T0229053

Perforator Flaps

Guest Editor

PETER C. NELIGAN, MB, BCh, FRCS(I), FRCS(C), FACS

CLINICS IN PLASTIC SURGERY

www.plasticsurgery.theclinics.com

October 2010 • Volume 37 • Number 4

SAUNDERS an imprint of ELSEVIER, Inc.

W.B. SAUNDERS COMPANY
A Division of Elsevier Inc.

1600 John F. Kennedy Boulevard ● Suite 1800 ● Philadelphia, Pennsylvania 19103-2899

http://www.theclinics.com

CLINICS IN PLASTIC SURGERY Volume 37, Number 4
October 2010 ISSN 0094-1298, ISBN-13: 978-1-4377-2486-8

Editor: Barbara Cohen-Kligerman

Clinics in Plastic Surgery (ISSN 0094-1298) is published quarterly by Elsevier Inc., 360 Park Avenue South, New York, NY 10010-1710. Months of issue are January, April, July, and October. Business and Editorial Offices: 1600 John F. Kennedy Blvd., Suite 1800, Philadelphia, PA 19103-2899. Periodicals postage paid at New York, NY and additional mailing offices. Subscription prices are $411.00 per year for US individuals, $617.00 per year for US institutions, $203.00 per year for US students and residents, $467.00 per year for Canadian individuals, $721.00 per year for Canadian institutions, $530.00 per year for international individuals, $721.00 per year for international institutions, and $256.00 per year for Canadian and foreign students/residents. To receive student/resident rate, orders must be accompanied by name of affiliated institution, date of term, and the *signature* of program/residency coordinator on institution letterhead. Orders will be billed at individual rate until proof of status is received. Foreign air speed delivery is included in all *Clinics* subscription prices. All prices are subject to change without notice. **POSTMASTER:** Send address changes to *Clinics in Plastic Surgery*, Elsevier Health Sciences Division, Subscription Customer Service, 3251 Riverport Lane, Maryland Heights, MO 63043. **Customer Service: 1-800-654-2452 (US and Canada). From outside of the United States and Canada, call 314-447-8871. Fax: 314-447-8029. E-mail: JournalsCustomerService-usa@elsevier.com (for print support); JournalsOnlineSupport-usa@elsevier.com (for online support).**

Reprints. For copies of 100 or more of articles in this publication, please contact the Commercial Reprints Department, Elsevier Inc., 360 Park Avenue South, New York, New York 10010-1710. Tel.: (+1) 212-633-3812; Fax: (+1) 212-462-1935; E-mail: reprints@elsevier.com.

Clinics in Plastic Surgery is covered in *Current Contents, EMBASE/Excerpta Medica, Science Citation Index, MEDLINE/ PubMed (Index Medicus), ASCA, and ISI/BIOMED.*

Printed and bound by CPI Group (UK) Ltd, Croydon, CR0 4YY

Transferred to Digital Print 2012

Contributors

GUEST EDITOR

PETER C. NELIGAN, MB, BCh, FRCS(I), ГПCS(C), ГAC3
Professor of Surgery and Director, Center for Reconstructive Surgery, University of Washington Medical Center, Seattle, Washington

AUTHORS

KHALID ALMUTARI, MD, MSc
Senior Plastic Surgery Resident, Department of Surgery, Dalhousie University, Halifax, Nova Scotia, Canada

PHILLIP N. BLONDEEL, MD, PhD, FCCP
Professor of Plastic Surgery, Department of Plastic and Reconstructive Surgery, University Hospital Gent, Gent, Belgium

RODNEY K. CHAN, MD
Chief Resident, Division of Plastic Surgery, Brigham and Women's Hospital, Boston, Massachusetts

ANNE DANCEY, MBChB, MmedSci, FRCS(Plast)
Microsurgery Fellow, Department of Plastic and Reconstructive Surgery, University Hospital Gent, Gent, Belgium

CHRISTOPHER GEDDES, MD, MS
Senior Orthopedic Resident, Department of Surgery, University of Toronto, Toronto, Ontario, Canada

GEOFFREY G. HALLOCK, MD
Division of Plastic Surgery, Sacred Heart Hospital; Division of Plastic Surgery, The Lehigh Valley Hospitals, Allentown; Division of Plastic Surgery, St Luke's Hospital, Bethlehem, Pennsylvania

MOUSTAPHA HAMDI, MD, PhD, FCCP
Professor in Plastic Surgery, Department of Plastic and Reconstructive Surgery, University Hospital Gent, Gent, Belgium

STEFAN O.P. HOFER, MD, PhD, FRCS(C)
Chief, Division of Plastic Surgery, Department of Surgery, University Health Network; Department of Surgical Oncology, University Health Network; Associate Professor and Wharton Chair in Reconstructive Plastic Surgery, University of Toronto, Toronto, Ontario, Canada

TAKUYA IIDA, MD
Assistant Professor, Plastic and Reconstructive Surgery, Graduate School of Medicine, University of Tokyo, Tokyo, Japan

ISAO KOSHIMA, MD
Assistant Professor, Plastic and Reconstructive Surgery, Graduate School of Medicine, University of Tokyo, Tokyo, Japan

DECLAN A. LANNON, MB, MSc, FRCS(Plast)
Consultant Plastic Surgeon, The Ulster Hospital, Dundonald, Belfast, Northern Ireland

JOAN E. LIPA, MD, MSc, FRCS(C), FACS
Associate Professor, Division of Plastic and Reconstructive Surgery, David Geffen School of Medicine, University of California Los Angeles, Los Angeles, California

DAVID W. MATHES, MD
Division of Plastic and Reconstructive Surgery, Department of Surgery, University of Washington School of Medicine, Seattle, Washington

MAKOTO MIHARA, MD
Assistant Professor, Plastic and
Reconstructive Surgery, Graduate School
of Medicine, University of Tokyo,
Tokyo, Japan

STEVEN F. MORRIS, MD, MSc, FRCSC
Professor of Surgery and Professor of
Anatomy, Department of Surgery, Dalhousie
University, Halifax, Nova Scotia, Canada

MARC A.M. MUREAU, MD, PhD
Assistant Professor and Head, Oncological
Reconstructive Surgery, Department of Plastic
and Reconstructive Surgery, Erasmus Medical
Center Rotterdam, Rotterdam,
The Netherlands

MITSUNAGA NARUSHIMA, MD
Assistant Professor, Plastic and
Reconstructive Surgery, Graduate School
of Medicine, University of Tokyo, Tokyo, Japan

**PETER C. NELIGAN, MB, BCh, FRCS(I),
FRCS(C), FACS**
Professor of Surgery and Director, Center
for Reconstructive Surgery, University
of Washington Medical Center,
Seattle, Washington

JULIAN J. PRIBAZ, MD
Professor of Surgery, Division of Plastic
Surgery, Brigham and Women's Hospital,
Boston, Massachusetts

MICHAEL SAUERBIER, MD, PhD
Department for Plastic, Hand and
Reconstructive Surgery, Main-Taunus
Hospitals GmbH, Academic Hospital University
of Frankfurt, Bad Soden am Taunus, Germany

FILIP B.J.L. STILLAERT, MD, FCCP
Resident, Department of Plastic and
Reconstructive Surgery, University Hospital
Gent, Gent, Belgium

MAOLIN TANG, MD
Professor and Chairman of Anatomy,
Department of Anatomy, Wenzhou Medical
College, Wenzhou University Town, Zhejiang,
People's Republic of China

**TIEW CHONG TEO, MD (Hons),
FRCS (Plast)**
Consultant Plastic and Reconstructive
Surgeon, Department of Plastic Surgery,
Queen Victoria Hospital, East Grinstead,
West Sussex, United Kingdom

CHARLES Y. TSENG, MD
Assistant Professor, Division of Plastic
and Reconstructive Surgery, David Geffen
School of Medicine, University of California
Los Angeles, Los Angeles, California

FRANK UNGLAUB, MD
Department for Plastic and Hand Surgery,
University Erlangen, Erlangen, Germany

TAKUMI YAMAMOTO, MD
Assistant Professor, Plastic and
Reconstructive Surgery, Graduate School
of Medicine, University of Tokyo, Tokyo, Japan

DAPING YANG, MD
Department of Plastic and Hand Surgery,
No. 2 Hospital of Harbin, Harbin,
People's Republic of China

Contents

Preface xi

Peter C. Neligan

The Anatomic Basis of Perforator Flaps 553

Steven F. Morris, Maolin Tang, Khalid Almutari, Christopher Geddes, and Daping Yang

The recent enthusiasm for perforator flaps underlines the need for a detailed understanding of the cutaneous vasculature. The principle determinant of success in perforator flap surgery is the inclusion of an adequately sized cutaneous perforator in the flap. Therefore, the size, distribution, and variability of cutaneous perforators of the human body are crucial to the design and execution of successful perforator flap surgery. Based on numerous anatomic studies, the authors have found that the main source arteries supplying the skin are fairly constant but the individual cutaneous perforators are quite variable. Knowledge of the overall architecture of the vasculature and an awareness of the variability, combined with a flexible operative plan, will enable the perforator flap surgeon to take advantage of the most appropriate perforators to execute a successful operative plan.

Where do Perforator Flaps Fit in our Armamentarium? 571

Julian J. Pribaz and Rodney K. Chan

This article reviews historical aspects of flap development, leading up to the exciting recognition of perforator flaps. The role and use of perforator-type flaps in the reconstructive armamentarium is reviewed as it pertains to different regions of the body.

Preoperative Imaging Techniques for Perforator Selection in Abdomen-Based Microsurgical Breast Reconstruction 581

David W. Mathes and Peter C. Neligan

The clinical application of perforator-based flaps for microsurgical breast reconstruction has increased exponentially over the past 10 years. The benefits of the procedure are thought to be that it produces less postoperative pain, lowers abdominal morbidity, and allows for better preservation of muscles at the donor site compared with conventional musculocutaneous flaps. The disadvantages of perforator flaps are that they are more difficult to harvest, which can result in a longer operative time and higher costs. The vascular anatomy of the deep inferior epigastric artery and its perforating branches in the abdominal wall varies greatly not only among individuals but also from one side of the abdomen to the other. Perforator location, number, caliber, and the intramuscular trajectory of the branches all impact the design and harvest of the flap. The creation of a presurgical map of the vessels on the abdomen can facilitate surgical planning and could decrease operating room time, reduce intraoperative complications, and lead to improved outcomes. This article reviews the available techniques for preoperative planning with the currently available imaging modalities: hand-held Doppler, color Doppler (duplex) ultrasound, CT angiography, and MR angiography.

Technical Tips for Safe Perforator Vessel Dissection Applicable to All Perforator Flaps 593

Anne Dancey and Phillip N. Blondeel

The introduction of perforator flaps by Koshima and Soeda in 1989 was met with much animosity in the surgical community. The flaps challenged conventional teaching and were often branded as being unsafe. Surgeries using perforator flaps are now routinely practiced all over the world, with increasing emphasis on minimizing donor site morbidity, and perforator flaps are becoming the current gold standard. The simple principles and techniques of perforator dissection can be applied to all perforator flaps, provided the surgeon has an intimate knowledge of the regional anatomy. Thus, virtually any piece of skin can be harvested as long as it incorporates a feeding vessel. This article highlights the essential techniques in planning and raising perforator flaps and the common pitfalls to be avoided.

The Integration of Muscle Perforator Flaps into a Community-Based Private Practice   607

Geoffrey G. Hallock

Over the past decade, muscle perforator flaps have proven their versatility as another important option when a soft tissue flap is essential. Valuable as either local or free flaps, these are no longer a novelty, and are perhaps even becoming a necessity for the mainstream reconstructive surgeon. Prior microsurgical capabilities will unquestionably simplify the transition to harvesting the diminutive vascular pedicle of these flaps, while perhaps shortening the learning curve, but these skills are not imperative. With proper assistance and perseverance, as with any other aspect of surgery, muscle perforator flaps can become a mainstay, if not the preferred method, for soft tissue repairs even in the community hospital where resources tend to be less available.

The Propeller Flap Concept   615

Tiew Chong Teo

The propeller flap, based on a single vascular pedicle supplying a fasciocutaneous island of skin, is a very useful technique to reconstruct soft tissue defects and has wide applications throughout the body. The use of this unique flap is pushing the boundaries of local flap reconstruction and bringing up intriguing questions about our understanding of the vascular basis of fasciocutaneous flaps.

Pedicled Perforator Flaps in the Head and Neck   627

Stefan O.P. Hofer and Marc A.M. Mureau

Perforator flaps, since their first description in 1989, have in many ways revolutionized reconstructive surgery. Whereas little more than a decade ago many surgeons were still hesitant to fully trust perforator flaps to be a reliable option, nowadays these flaps are often first choice. Investigators have to remain critical, however, of their advances and realize that not every reconstruction will require or benefit from a perforator flap, as previously well-established, nonperforator flaps still have their indication and can give excellent results. The most important skill in reconstructive surgery of the head and neck is not cutting the flap but assessing the defect, planning the reconstruction, and choosing wisely from the ever-increasing options available.

Perforator Flaps in Breast Reconstruction   641

Charles Y. Tseng and Joan E. Lipa

Patients are well informed and seek autogenous breast reconstruction. The motivating factors include a preference for autologous tissue reconstruction and the complementary improvement in body contour, safety concerns surrounding implants, and implant-related complications in the setting of previous radiation therapy. In this article a variety of perforator flaps from donor sites that include the trunk (thoraco-dorsal artery perforator and intercostal artery perforator), abdomen (deep inferior epigastric artery perforator and superficial inferior epigastric artery), and buttock (superior gluteal artery perforator and inferior gluteal artery perforator) are described. Flaps from the trunk can be pedicled for partial breast reconstruction, and free flaps from the other donor sites can completely restore a natural-looking breast. The information obtained from preoperative CT and MRI can direct the surgeon toward the most successful operative plan. However, the decision as to which flap may be most appropriate for an individual patient is complex. This article reviews pertinent surgical anatomy, preoperative planning, intraoperative decision making in flap elevation, and reported outcomes.

Pedicled Perforator Flaps in the Trunk   655

Moustapha Hamdi and Filip B.J.L. Stillaert

Trunk defects can be approached through a multitude of regional flaps that can be harvested from the shoulder girdle, the epigastric axis, the paraspinal region, or the pelvic girdle. The aim of the reconstruction is to provide adequate and tension-free restoration of tissue integrity with minimal functional morbidity, water- and airtight closure of cavities, and coverage of exposed vital structures. Potential donor sites should be estimated for their tissue quality and anticipated donor site morbidity. The prototypical pedicled flap has a constant, reliable anatomy; however, the pedicled flap should have a configuration that is versatile and adequate for coverage and should resist infection. Also, the surgical technique should be uncomplicated.

Perforator Flaps in the Upper Extremity   667

Michael Sauerbier and Frank Unglaub

Perforator flaps are frequently used for defect coverage for the whole body. There are strong indications for the use of perforator flaps in the upper extremity. This article demonstrates the possibilities for defect coverage with perforator flaps as well as their anatomic and technical considerations. Lateral arm, posterior interosseous artery, ulnar artery, radial artery perforator flaps, and intrinsic hand flaps are described.

Versatility of the Pedicled Anterolateral Thigh Flap   677

Peter C. Neligan and Declan A. Lannon

The pedicled anterolateral thigh flap is a useful addition to our armamentarium. It provides excellent cover for defects in the lower abdomen, pelvis, and perineum. It also has the added advantage of not sacrificing any muscle, thereby minimizing the risk for donor morbidity. This article reviews the major applications of the proximally pedicled anterolateral thigh flap, describes the technique of flap harvest, and discusses techniques of flap transposition as well as pointing out some potential hazards.

Perforator Flaps and Supermicrosurgery   683

Isao Koshima, Takumi Yamamoto, Mitsunaga Narushima, Makoto Mihara, and Takuya Iida

The introduction of supermicrosurgery, which allows the anastomosis of smaller caliber vessels and microvascular dissection of vessels ranging from 0.3 to 0.8 mm in diameter, has led to the development of new reconstructive techniques. New applications of this technique are for crushed fingertip replantations with venule grafts, toe tip transfers for fingertip loss, partial auricular transfers for total tracheal and eyelid defects, and lymphaticovenular anastomoses under local anesthesia for lymphedema. Regarding free flaps, free perforator-to-perforator flaps, including deep inferior epigastric perforator or paraumbilical perforator flaps, gluteal artery perforator flaps, thoracodorsal artery perforator flaps, anterolateral thigh perforator flaps, superficial circumflex iliac artery perforator flaps, tensor fasciae lata perforator flaps, and medial plantar perforator flaps, with a short pedicle, have been used for extremity and facial defects. The success rate is almost the same as that of usual free flap transfers with large and long pedicles. The advantages of these flaps are the simple operation and the short time needed for flap elevation, plus the fact that the flaps can be obtained from anywhere in concealed areas. The disadvantages are the need for supermicrosurgical technique and the anatomic variation of these perforators.

Index   **691**

Clinics in Plastic Surgery

FORTHCOMING ISSUES

January 2010

Vascular Anomalies
Chad Perlyn, MD, PhD,
and Arin K. Greene, MD, MMSc,
Guest Editors

April 2011

**Cosmetic Medicine and Minimally Invasive
Surgery/State of the Art**
Malcolm D. Paul, MD, FACS,
Raffi Hovsepian, MD, and
Adam Rotunda, MD, *Guest Editors*

July 2011

Toolbox for Autologous Breast Reconstruction
Maurice Nahabedian, MD,
Guest Editor

RECENT ISSUES

July 2010

Abdominoplasty
Al Aly, MD, FACS,
Guest Editor

April 2010

Rhinoplasty: Current Concepts
Ronald P. Gruber, MD, and
David Stepnick, MD, FACS,
Guest Editors

January 2010

Cutaneous Melanoma
William Dzwierzynski, MD, FACS,
Guest Editor

ISSUES OF RELATED INTEREST

Facial Plastic Surgery Clinics of North America August 2010 (Vol. 18, No. 3)
Periocular Rejuvenation
Edward H. Farrior, MD, *Guest Editor*
Available at: http://www.facialplastic.theclinics.com/

Oral and Maxillofacial Surgery Clinics of North America February 2010 (Vol. 22, No. 1)
Clinical Innovation and Technology in Craniomaxillofacial Surgery
Bernard J. Costello, DMD, MD, *Guest Editor*
Available at: http://www.oralmaxsurgery.theclinics.com/

THE CLINICS ARE NOW AVAILABLE ONLINE!

Access your subscription at:
www.theclinics.com

Preface

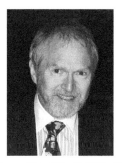

Peter C. Neligan, MB, BCh, FRCS(I), FRCS(C), FACS
Guest Editor

When I was first exposed to the concept of perforator flaps, I did not immediately embrace the idea. In fact, I was hard pressed to see the point. From my perspective, I couldn't understand why one would jeopardize the vascularity of a flap by dissecting its major pedicle to an extent that I had always been taught was dangerous. I had been taught to sew the skin paddle of any flap to the underlying muscle so as not to risk shearing the perforating vessels supplying the skin from within the muscle. These myocutaneous flaps were reliable; the anatomy was well known, and they were safe. Why in the world would I take such a risk and make a perfectly safe flap an unsafe one? One day I was doing a free TRAM flap and I decided, out of curiosity, to look at the perforators on the nonpedicled side. I came upon a very large perforator and before I knew it I had dissected my first DIEAP flap. Since then, I have come to appreciate the versatility of perforator flaps and have recognized how much they add to our reconstructive ability.

Perforator flaps are no longer new. In fact this is the second issue of *Clinics in Plastic Surgery* to be devoted to perforator flaps. However, it is surprising that many people are scared by the concept and haven't embraced this new technique of flap harvest—for that's what it is, a technique. It is also curious that in some parts of the world perforator flaps are more widely used than in others. For example, their use in Europe is far more common than their use in North America. Similarly, perforator flaps are more commonly used in some anatomic regions than in others. The use of DIEAP flaps in postmastectomy breast reconstruction is a case in point. However, even in the breast, the majority of plastic surgeons, at least in North America, are not using them. Interestingly, use of perforator flaps in breast reconstruction is being driven, at least to some extent, by the patient. I regularly have women show up to my clinic specifically to enquire about DIEAP flap breast reconstruction. This seems to be unique to the breast, and we do not see it in other sites.

In this issue I have asked the leaders in this field to bring us up-to-date on the latest developments in perforator flaps: what works, what doesn't work, and how to make them safer. I hope you find this a useful issue.

Peter C. Neligan, MB, BCh, FRCS(I), FRCS(C), FACS
University of Washington Medical Center
Division of Plastic Surgery
Box 356410
1959 NE Pacific Street
Seattle, WA 98195-6410, USA

E-mail address:
pneligan@u.washington.edu

Clin Plastic Surg 37 (2010) xi
doi:10.1016/j.cps.2010.07.002
0094-1298/10/$ – see front matter

The Anatomic Basis of Perforator Flaps

Steven F. Morris, MD, MSc, FRCSC[a],*, Maolin Tang, MD[b],
Khalid Almutari, MD, MSc[c], Christopher Geddes, MD, MS[d],
Daping Yang, MD[e]

KEYWORDS

- Perforator flap surgery • Cutaneous vasculature • Anatomy
- Reconstructive plastic surgery

The vascular anatomy of cutaneous perforators is of vital importance for the design of successful perforator flaps. The detailed knowledge of this vascular anatomy provides the framework for flap elevation. Therefore, it is critical that the reconstructive surgeon has a detailed understanding of the vascular anatomy of the human integument. The purpose of this article is to provide an overview of the vascular anatomy of the human body to allow surgeons to use and customize perforator flaps in reconstructive plastic surgery.

HISTORICAL PERSPECTIVE

Harvey, in the 1600s, and Thomas and Spalteholz, in the 1800s, provided some of the earliest descriptions of the cutaneous vasculature.[1] In the late 1880s, Carl Manchot[2] performed a detailed study of the human cutaneous blood supply (**Fig. 1**) and provided an early description of the vascular territories of the human body. This work was done by dissection alone, which is a remarkable feat given the complexity of the human skin vasculature. Manchot's description of the cutaneous vasculature, and in particular the vascular territories of the integument, has stood the test

of time. In the 1930s, Michel Salmon[3] did a series of anatomic dissections using the original lead oxide injection technique and provided the earliest and detailed descriptions of the vascular supply to the skin (**Fig. 2**). He contributed important concepts regarding the vasculature that remain relevant to the reconstructive surgeon, including observations about the pattern of cutaneous perforators. Subsequently, Ian Taylor and Palmer[4] have provided comprehensive vascular studies of the human integument and together with John Palmer described the angiosomes of the body (**Fig. 3**). The angiosome concept provided an important early framework for the development of perforator flaps. The use of the Doppler was described to identify the variable skin perforators. More recently, anatomic techniques have included a combination of vascular injection studies and three-dimensional (3D) computerized angiography to provide the most detailed illustrations of the vascular anatomy of the integument.[5–7] The lead oxide injection technique was initially described by Michel Salmon[3] in the 1930s. Rees and Taylor[8] modified the technique and used it extensively in a series of anatomic projects.[9] The authors have used this technique to comprehensively document the human cutaneous perforators.[10–13]

[a] Department of Surgery, Dalhousie University, 4443-1796 Summer Street, Halifax, Nova Scotia, Canada B3H 3A7
[b] Department of Anatomy, Wenzhou Medical College, Wenzhou University Town, Zhejiang 325000, PR. China
[c] Department of Surgery, Dalhousie University, Canada
[d] Department of Surgery, University of Toronto, Canada
[e] Department of Plastic and Hand Surgery, No 2 Hospital of Harbin, Harbin 150086, PR China
* Corresponding author.
E-mail address: sfmorris@dal.ca

Clin Plastic Surg 37 (2010) 553–570
doi:10.1016/j.cps.2010.06.006
0094-1298/10/$ – see front matter © 2010 Elsevier Inc. All rights reserved.

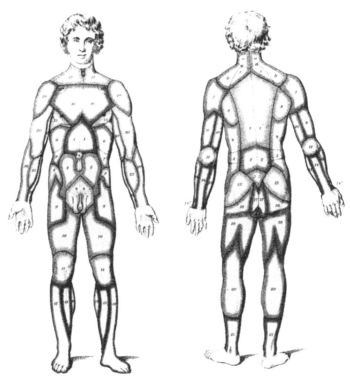

Fig. 1. The vascular territories of the human body by Carl Manchot. Manchot described the vascular territories of the human body based on dissection of the cutaneous vessels in the 1880s. (*From* Morris SF, Miller B, Taylor GI. In: Blondeel PN, Morris SF, Hallock GG, et al, editors. Perforator flaps, anatomy, technique and clinical applications. St Louis (MO): Quality Medical Publishing; 2006. Fig. 2–1, p. 15; Fig. 2–8, p. 31, Chapter 2; with permission.)

CURRENT ANATOMIC TECHNIQUE

The authors have further modified the lead oxide injection technique to optimize 3-D angiography.[14,15] The volume of lead oxide has been minimized and the gelatin modified to improve the CT images. The injection studies are performed on fresh cadavers following university ethical guidelines. Bony landmarks are marked with lead wire and then photographs and measurements are taken. The cadaver is injected through the femoral vessels using 100 g per 100 mL of lead oxide, gelatin, and water solution for a total infusing volume of 25 mL per kilogram (**Fig. 4**). The injectant is warmed to 40°C. After injection, the cadaver is cooled to 4° for 24 hours and then a CT scan and dissection are performed. Depending on the specific study, the skin incisions will vary, but a sequential dissection technique is usually used. Dissection notes are taken on specific perforators and they are marked with radio opaque beads. Dissection notes are compared with the CT images of the cadaver injection and the source of vessels is identified.

Radiography is used for all dissected structures and then the data regarding the perforator diameter, length, source vessel, and branches are recorded. These are compared with the 3-D images from CT scans.

THREE-DIMENSIONAL ANATOMIC TECHNIQUE

The two-dimensional angiographic images can create confusing superimposed angiograms that can be difficult to interpret to assess the 3-D position and the relationship of vessels to other structures.[5] The authors use angiography and Materialise's Interactive Medical Image Control System (Mimics) to create a 3-D model of the anatomy of the area of interest.[5–7] The 3-D microvascular images prepared by whole-body radio opaque medium injection and processed using the Mimics software package can be used to design a specific flap. Using this technique, the bone, soft tissue, skin, and vascular structures can be demonstrated in a layer-by-layer transparent process (**Fig. 5**). The detailed views of the

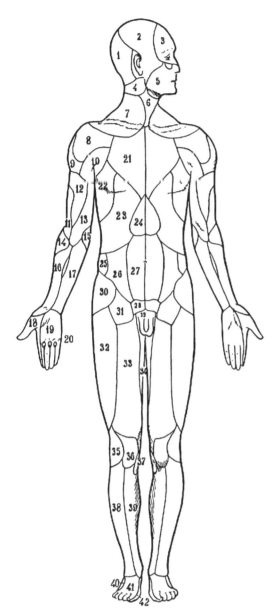

Fig. 2. Michel Salmon's vascular territories of the body. (*From* Taylor GI, Ives A, Dhar S. Vascular territories. In: Mathes SJ, editor. Plastic surgery. 2nd edition, vol. 1. Philadelphia: Elsevier; 2006 . p. 321, Fig. 15.4; with permission.)

microvasculature provide extensive information regarding the course of vessels in all layers of tissue.

After the cadaver vascular injection is completed, cadavers are imaged by a CT scanner (General Electric Lightspeed H16; General Electric Medical Systems, Milwaukee, WI, USA) and the data are transferred to a computer. Mimics interactively reads CT and MRI data in the Digital Imaging and Communications in Medicine

(DICOM) format. Segmentation and editing tools enable the user to manipulate the data to select the specific tissue type required (eg, bone, soft tissue, skin and vessels) (see **Fig. 5**). Once an area of interest is separated, it can be visualized in 3D. After visualization, a file can be made to interface with STL or MedCAD (Materialise Group, Leuven, Belgium) data imported as STL files or can be visualized in 3D for design validation based on the anatomic geometry. It is possible for a surgeon to perform data analysis, plan and simulate surgical procedures, and make critical decisions on approaches to surgery using Mimics software.

The threshold of the data set is manipulated to obtain the best visual image of the vascular anatomy. In order to show different vascular density, the threshold unit can be adjusted; the lower the threshold the more vascular density (**Fig. 6**). Because other structures, such as bone, have a density similar to the lead-filled arteries (see **Fig. 6**C), further manipulation is made to physically or digitally remove these structures to improve the clarity of the blood vessels. After these procedures, a 3-D reconstruction of the vasculature, which can be viewed stereoscopically, is generated. The same process is repeated for the 3-D reconstruction of the overlying skin vascular perforators (**Fig. 7**) and the underlying bone structure (**Fig. 8**). This technique allows the demonstration of the fine details of the course of arteries, and their 3-D relationship to surrounding structures and location.

THREE-DIMENSIONAL ANATOMY OF THE PERFORATOR FLAPS

The 3-D models of individual perforator flaps demonstrate the flap source artery, its course, distribution, and anastomosis with adjacent arteries (see **Figs. 5–7**). **Fig. 7**A shows the transverse branch of the deep circumflex iliac artery (DCIA) as it anastomoses with the anterior branch of the lumbar artery and sends a cutaneous perforator to the skin. **Fig. 7**B shows the anastomoses within the deep inferior epigastric perforator flap. A transparent image can be created that shows the direction and location of source arteries within each layer of a perforator flap (see **Fig. 7**A). Using the tools, dynamic region growing or edit mask in 3D, the authors can show a source artery and each perforator (**Fig. 9**).

There are several advantages of 3-D reconstruction by Mimics using the whole-cadaver radiographic medium injection technique:

1. Flap design after whole-body angiography and 3-D reconstruction is superior to individual flap dissection with isolated injection.

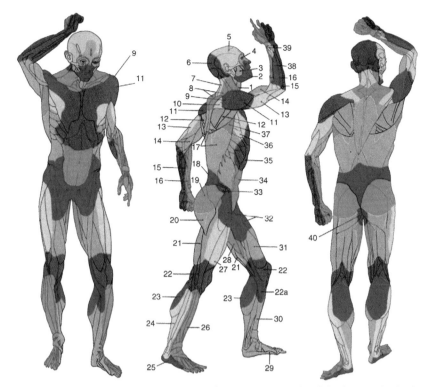

Fig. 3. G. Ian Taylor's vascular territories, angiosomes of the source vessels of the human body. (*From* Taylor GI, Ives A, Dhar S. Vascular territories. In: Mathes SJ, editor. Plastic surgery. 2nd edition, vol. 1. Philadelphia: Elsevier; 2006. p. 321, Fig. 15.4; with permission.)

2. 3-D visualization of vascular anatomy by whole-body angiography CT scan produces a complete data set so that layer-by-layer information exists to identify the location of each individual source artery with its course, direction, and anastomosis with other vessels. It is therefore helpful for overall anatomic analysis.

3. This technique allows dissection of the cadaver after 3-D reconstruction to correlate with the 3-D images.

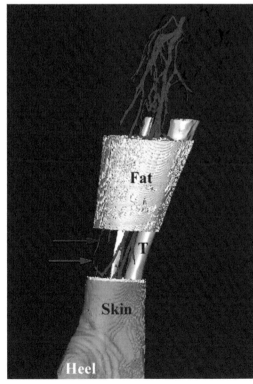

Fig. 5. Posterior view: 3-D reconstruction of the leg. Blue arrow shows a descending perforator; pink arrow points to the ascending branch of peroneal artery perforator. T, tibia.

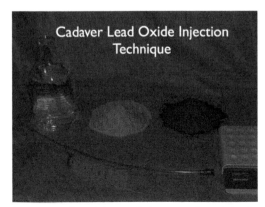

Fig. 4. Lead oxide, gelatin vascular injection technique.

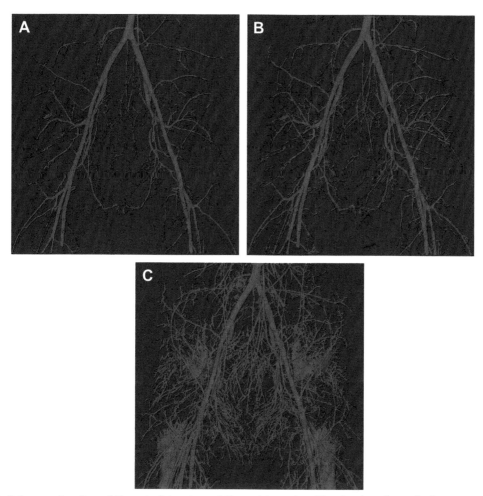

Fig. 6. 3-D reconstruction of the arterial system of the pelvic region. The density of vessels changes with the threshold of the data set: (*A*) 2500–2976; (*B*) 1800–2976; (*C*) 1000–2976 (some compact bone has similar density to the injected arteries).

4. After whole-body angiographic injection, the arteries are marked by lead oxide in the series of CT images. The image capture, reorganization, and correlation with the microvasculature are therefore straight forward using the Mimics process. Visible human or uninjected living-person CT images are difficult to recognize and match the microvascular network by 3-D programs.

OVERVIEW OF THE PERFORATORS OF THE BODY

Based on numerous cadaver injection studies the authors have described the cutaneous perforators of the human body.[10–13] These perforators are shown diagrammatically in **Fig. 10** and abbreviations for the Fig. are shown in **Table 1**. The various

vascular territories are shown in different colors to highlight the zones of vasculature of the major source vessels. Within each vascular territory, a variable number of cutaneous perforators supply the skin. These can be easily dissected and described in a cadaver. In preoperative patients at the time of perforator flap planning, the overall pattern of perforator position is taken into consideration with either Doppler study or CT angiographic study of the actual perforator position and size. The source vessels that supply the perforators to the skin are the named main vessels in each anatomic region. These become the source vessel for the individual perforator flap. For example, the perforators for the anterolateral thigh flap (descending branch of the lateral circumflex femoral artery perforator flap), are generally located around the midpoint of the thigh between the anterior superior iliac spine

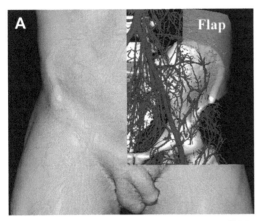

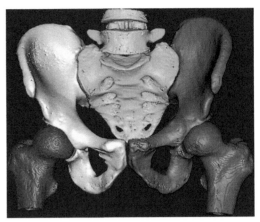

Fig. 8. 3-D reconstruction of the bones of the pelvis. This image is obtained by subtracting the other tissues away from the 3-D image shown in **Fig. 7**.

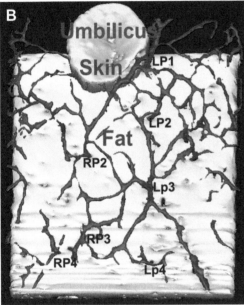

Fig. 7. (*A*) 3-D reconstruction to demonstrate a deep circumflex iliac artery (DCIA) osteocutaneous perforator flap. This specimen is the same as shown in **Fig. 6**. (*B*) 3-D reconstruction of abdominal perforator from deep inferior epigastric artery (DIEA). It is a female specimen. Reading down from umbilicus: LP1–4, left DIEA perforators; RP2–4, right DIEA perforators; (RP1 hidden in umbilicus). Frequently, they are true anastomoses with no change in caliber between left and right deep inferior epigastric perforator (DIEAP), crossing the midline.

and the lateral edge of the patella. The individual perforators are quite variable in size and exact position, but generally the perforators of each source vessel supply a specified region of the skin of the body.

The route of perforators to skin may be in one of three general patterns: (1) directly from source vessels to the skin, running along the skin for long distances as axial vessels; (2) septocutaneous vessels that pass through septa from source

vessels to the skin; and (3) musculocutaneous perforators that arise from source vessels and penetrate a muscle before supplying the skin. Almost all of these perforators may be variable. The exact terminology of the specific perforator to the skin is disputed somewhat but it is agreed that flap survival is not influenced by the specific source of the perforator to skin but rather the caliber and course of the vessel. The direction and pattern of skin supply of an individual perforator will have an effect on flap viability.[16] Many classifications have been applied to the perforators of the skin, however, it is unimportant what the perforator is called as long as it is of sufficient caliber to provide adequate vascularization of the perforator flap. There are a limited number of source vessels in the body and these supply perforators to the skin in a somewhat predictable but variable manner. Salmon noted that vessels supply vascular branches to each structure that they pass and this is certainly true in the authors' anatomic dissections.[3]

CUTANEOUS VASCULATURE OF THE HEAD AND NECK

In the skin of the head and neck, an abundance of arteries interconnects to form a rich network, particularly in the face and scalp (**Fig. 11**). Branches of the external carotid system, the transverse cervical or the suprascapular artery, supply most of the head and neck skin, with the exception of an area that surrounds the eyes and covers the central forehead and upper two-thirds of the nose (see **Fig. 11**). There is a rich midline network of vessels in the forehead and nose provided by branches of the internal carotid system, which link the facial and superficial temporal arteries of

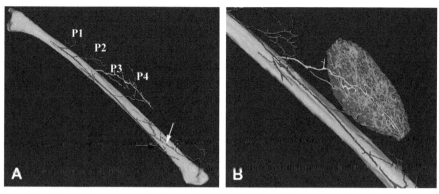

Fig. 9. 3-D reconstruction of the peroneal artery and fibula. (*A*) Shows the peroneal perforators (P1–P4), posterior branch of the lateral malleolus (*yellow arrow*), and posterior communicating branches (*blue arrow*). (*B*) Peroneal perforator flap.

either side as an arcade. The cutaneous perforators radiate from fixed points, either from bony foramina or from sites where the deep fascia is attached to bone. They connect with their opposite artery across the midline to form vascular arches. The connections often consist of reduced-caliber choke arteries, but frequently they are true anastomoses with no change in caliber between vascular territories. The vascularity of the face and scalp is rich and there are numerous perforator flap options (as shown in Dr Hofer's article elsewhere in this issue).

The perforators supplying the skin of the neck pierce the cervical fascia and branch to form

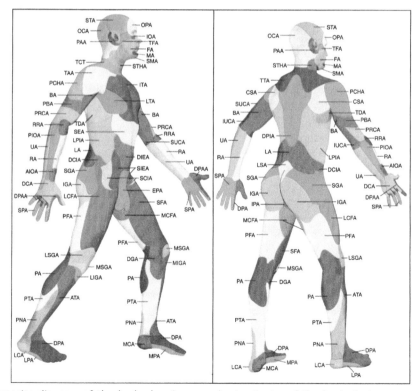

Fig. 10. Composite diagram of the body showing vascular territories of the body that correspond to source arteries that supply musculocutaneous or septocutaneous perforators to the integument. Anterior interosseous artery. See **Table 1** for an explanation of the abbreviations. (*From* Morris SF, Miller B, Taylor GI. In: Blondeel PN, Morris SF, Hallock GG, et al, editors. Perforator flaps, anatomy, technique and clinical applications. St Louis (MO): Quality Medical Publishing; 2006. Fig. 2–1, p. 15; Fig. 2–8, p. 31, Chapter 2; with permission.)

Table 1
Vascular territories

Artery	Artery Abbreviation
Anterior interosseous artery	AIOA
Anterior tibial artery	ATA
Brachial artery	BA
Circumflex scapular artery	CSA
Deep circumflex iliac artery	DCIA
Deep inferior epigastric artery	DIEA
Deep palmar arch	DPAA
Descending genicular artery	DGA
Dorsal branch of posterior intercostal artery	DP1A
Dorsal carpal arch	DCA
Dorsal pedis artery	DPA
External pudendal artery	EPA
Facial artery	FA
Mental artery	MA
Submental artery	SMA
Inferior gluteal artery	IGA
Inferior ulnar collateral artery	IUCA
Infraorbital artery	IOA
Internal pudendal arteries	IPA
Internal thoracic (mammary) artery	ITA
Lateral branches of posterior intercostal artery	LPIA
Lateral calcaneal artery	LCA
Lateral circumflex femoral artery	LCFA
Lateral inferior genicular artery	LIGA
Lateral plantar artery	LPA
Lateral sacral arteries	LSA
Lateral superior genicular artery	LSGA
Lateral thoracic (mammary) artery	LTA
Lumbar arteries	LA
Medial calcaneal artery	MCA
Medial circumflex femoral artery	MCFA
Medial inferior genicular artery	MIGA
Medial superior genicular artery	MSGA
Occipital artery	OCA
Ophthalmic artery	OPA
Peroneal artery	PNA
Popliteal artery	PA
Lateral sural artery	LSA
Medial sural artery	MSA
Posterior auricular artery	PAURA
Posterior circumflex humeral artery	PCHA
Posterior interosseous artery	PIOA
Posterior radial collateral artery	PRCA
Posterior tibial artery	PTA
Profunda brachial artery	PBA
Profunda femoris artery	PFA

(*continued on next page*)

Table 1
(continued)

Artery	Artery Abbreviation
Radial artery	RA
Radial recurrent artery	RRA
Superficial circumflex iliac artery	SCIA
Superficial femoral artery	SFA
Superficial inferior epigastric artery	SIEA
Superficial palmar arch	SPA
Superficial temporal artery	STA
Superior epigastric artery-	SEA
Superior gluteal artery	SGA
Superior thyroid artery	STHA
Superior ulnar collateral artery	SUCA
Thoracoacromial artery	TAA
Thoracodorsal artery	TDA
Thyrocervical trunk	TCT
Dorsal scapular artery	DSA
Suprascapular artery	SSA
Transverse cervical artery	TCA
Transverse facial artery	TFA
Ulnar artery	UA

From Morris SF, Miller B, Taylor GI. In: Blondeel PN, Morris SF, Hallock GG, et al, editors. Perforator flaps, anatomy, technique and clinical applications. St Louis (MO): Quality Medical Publishing; 2006. Fig. 2–1, p. 15; Fig. 2–8, p. 31, Chapter 2; with permission.

a rich plexus across the neck that overflows onto the adjacent chest, shoulder, and back. The branches of these cutaneous perforators are intimately related to the undersurface and substance of the platysma muscle, which they perforate to supply the subdermal plexus.

The head and neck compose the smallest region of the body and have approximately 25 perforators greater than 0.5 mm diameter. The vascular supply to the integument of the head and neck is from the terminal cutaneous vessels of 10 source arteries comprising the vascular territories in this region.[10] The large caliber and superficial nature of the vessels in this region can be attributed to the overlay of the facial and scalp skin on the bony skeleton of the head. In contrast, the longitudinal muscle structure of the neck allows for smaller, more numerous musculocutaneous perforators to supply the skin in this region. The average diameter and area supplied by a single perforator are approximately 0.9 mm and 32 cm², respectively.

CUTANEOUS VASCULATURE OF THE UPPER EXTREMITY

The vascular supply to the integument of the upper extremity is from the axillary artery and its terminal branches (**Fig. 12**). The individual cutaneous perforators tend to cluster around the major named source vessels shown in **Fig. 12**. The brachial artery begins at the lower border of the teres major muscle as the continuation of the axillary artery and runs down the medial aspect of the arm and divides into the radial and ulnar arteries in the cubital fossa. The radial and ulnar arteries and the anterior and posterior interosseous arteries supply the forearm. The palmar aspect of the hand is supplied predominantly by the ulnar artery through the superficial palmar arch. The dorsum is supplied by the radial artery through the dorsal metacarpal arteries. The digital arteries arising from the arches in the hand supply the fingers and thumb. The size of the vascular territories in the upper limb is larger proximally and becomes progressively smaller distally. In the upper arm and in the proximal part of the forearm, the perforators are predominantly musculocutaneous and in the distal forearm, septocutaneous

An average of 48 perforators in 15 vascular territories supply the integument of the upper extremity (**Fig. 13**).[11] Each territory is supplied by a named source artery that provides a variable number of cutaneous perforators. The precise location and number of perforators in each

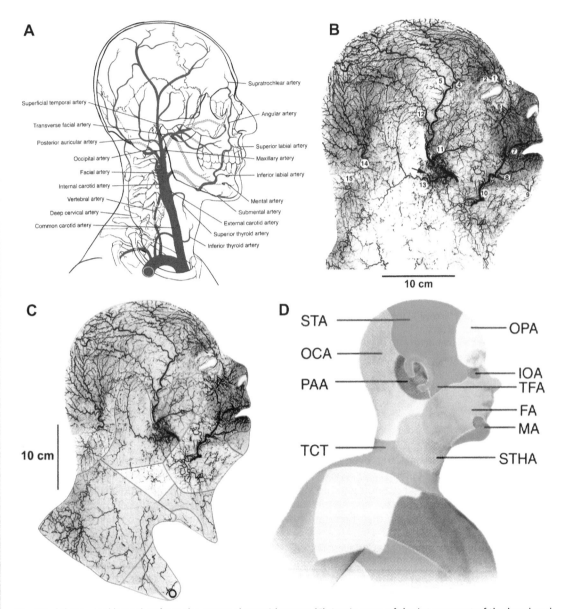

Fig. 11. (*A*) Principal branches from the external carotid artery. (*B*) Angiogram of the integument of the head and neck: 1, supratrochlear artery; 2, supraorbital artery; 3, dorsal nasal artery; 4, frontal branch of superficial temporal artery; 5, parietal branch of superficial temporal artery; 6, infraorbital artery; 7, superior labial artery; 8, inferior labial artery; 9, mental artery; 10, facial artery; 11, transverse facial artery; 12, superior auricular artery; 13, posterior auricular artery; 14, occipital artery; 15, descending branch of the occipital artery. (*C*) Vascular territories of the integument of the head and neck. O, acromion. (*D*) The vascular territories of the integument of the head and neck. FA, facial artery; IOA, infraorbital artery; MA, mental artery; OCA, occipital artery; PAA, posterior auricular artery; STA, superficial temporal artery; STHA, superior thyroid artery; TCT, thyrocervical trunk; TFA, transverse facial artery. (*From* Yang D, Tang M, Geddes CR, et al. Anatomy of the integument of the head and neck. In: Blondeel PN, Morris SF, Hallock GG, et al, editors. Perforator flaps, anatomy, technique and clinical applications. St. Louis (MO): Quality Medical Publishing; 2006. Fig. 8.4, p. 138; with permission.)

territory are quite variable. Despite this variability between individual perforators, the cutaneous areas or vascular territories supplied by the source vessels are uniform. Musculocutaneous perforators are more numerous in the upper arm and proximal forearm. Septocutaneous arteries predominated in the shoulder, elbow, distal forearm, and hand regions. The average perforator in the upper extremity is approximately 0.7 mm in diameter and supplies an average of 35 cm[2].[11]

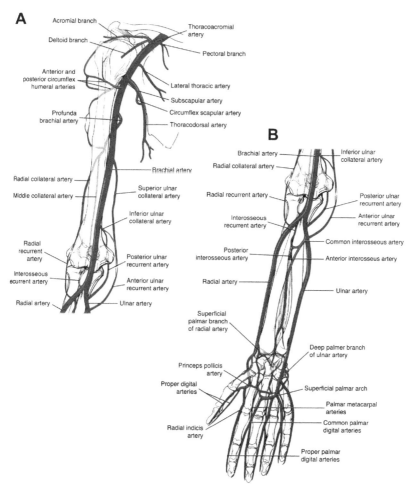

Fig. 12. (*A, B*) Arteries of the upper extremity. (*From* Thomas B, Geddes CR, Tang M, et al. In: Blondeel PN, Morris SF, Hallock GG, et al, editors. Perforator flaps, anatomy, technique and clinical applications. St Louis (MO): Quality Medical Publishing; 2006. Fig. 12–1, p. 221, Chapter 12; with permission.)

Perforator flaps that are particularly useful and commonly used include those that are based on perforators of the posterior radial collateral artery (lateral arm flap), anterior and posterior interosseous arteries (posterior interosseous flap), radial artery, ulnar artery, and dorsal carpal arch (dorsal metacarpal artery flap). (See Dr Sauerbier's article on perforator flaps in the upper extremity). Vessels in the hand can be used in a great variety of ways to create useful flaps for hand reconstruction (**Fig. 14**).

CUTANEOUS VASCULATURE OF THE TRUNK

The integument of the trunk is used extensively in reconstructive surgery for flap harvest. Large vascular perforators from 15 source arteries supply the various donor sites of the trunk.[12] The majority of these perforators are musculocutaneous, originating from the primary blood supply supplying the broad superficial muscles in this region. Several large septocutaneous perforators arise from the perimeter of these muscles and from near the joint creases of the extremities where the skin is tethered to underlying connective tissue. The perforators to the skin of the trunk are shown in **Figs. 15–17**. There are numerous larger perforators that can be used for pedicled or free flap harvest. The large septocutaneous perforators are easily distinguishable in angiograms of the integument because they frequently have a larger diameter and travel greater distances, thus supplying large vascular territories. For example, the lateral thoracic artery, the second and third anterior intercostals, the superficial inferior epigastric, and superficial circumflex femoral arteries all emerge as septocutaneous perforators and travel long distances in the skin.

The arterial blood supply of the trunk arises from 3 primary arterial systems: the subclavian/axillary

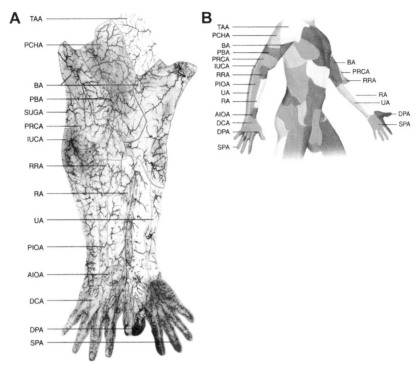

Fig. 13. (*A*) Angiogram of the integument of the upper extremity of a human cadaver. (*B*) Vascular territories of the integument of the upper extremity of a human cadaver. AIOA, anterior interosseous artery; BA, brachial artery; DCA, dorsal carpal arch; DPA, deep palmer arch; IUCA, inferior ulnar collateral artery; PBA, profunda brachial artery; PCHA, posterior circumflex humeral artery; PIOA, posterior interosseous artery; PRCA, posterior radial collateral artery; RA, radial artery; RRA, radial recurrent artery; SPA, superior palmer arch; SUCA, superior ulnar collateral artery; TAA, thoracoacromial artery; UA, ulnar artery. (*From* Thomas B, Geddes CR, Tang M, et al. In: Blondeel PN, Morris SF, Hallock GG, et al, editors. Perforator flaps, anatomy, technique and clinical applications. St Louis (MO): Quality Medical Publishing; 2006. Fig. 12–1, p. 221, Chapter 12; with permission.)

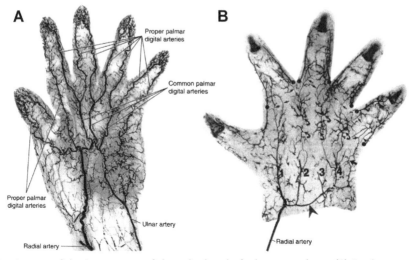

Fig. 14. (*A*) Angiogram of the integument of the volar hand of a human cadaver. (*B*) Angiogram of the integument of the dorsal hand of a human cadaver. The dorsal carpal arch (*Large arrow*) supplies 4 dorsal metacarpal arteries (1–4). The curved arrows mark the dorsal perforators of the palmer digital arteries. (*From* Thomas B, Geddes CR, Tang M, et al. In: Blondeel PN, Morris SF, Hallock GG, et al, editors. Perforator flaps, anatomy, technique and clinical applications. St Louis (MO): Quality Medical Publishing; 2006. Fig. 12–1, p. 221, Chapter 12; with permission.)

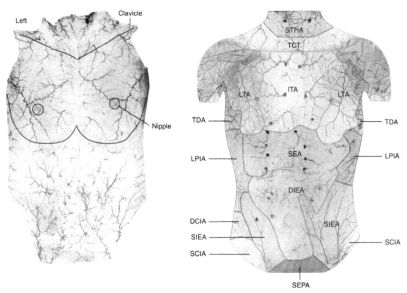

Fig. 15. Angiogram of the integument of the anterior trunk. Overlying lead wires mark out the clavicles, nipples, and inframammary creases. On the right, the colored vascular territories of the various source vessels are shown. DCIA, deep circumflex iliac artery; DIEA, deep inferior epigastric artery; LPIA, lateral posterior intercostal arteries; LTA, lateral thoracic artery; SCIA, superficial circumflex iliac artery; SEA, superior epigastric artery; SEPA, superficial external pudendal artery; SIEA, superficial inferior epigastric artery; STHA, superior thyroid artery; TCT, Thyrocervical trunk; TDA, thoracodorsal artery; ITA, internal thoracic artery; (*From* Geddes CR, Tang M, Yang D, et al. In: Blondeel PN, Morris SF, Hallock GG, et al, editors. Perforator flaps, anatomy, technique and clinical applications. St Louis (MO): Quality Medical Publishing; 2006. Fig. 18–3, p. 365, Chapter 18; with permission.)

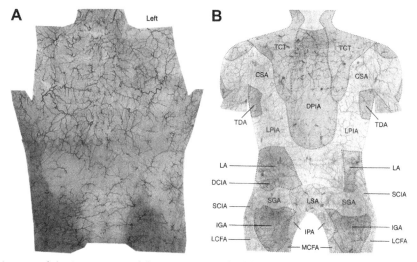

Fig. 16. Angiogram of the integument of the posterior trunk. (*A*) Angiogram. (*B*) Colored vascular territories of the various source vessels are shown. CSA, circumflex scapular artery; DCIA, deep circumflex iliac artery; DPIA, dorsal posterior intercostal arteries; IGA, inferior gluteal arteries; IPA, internal pudendal artery; LA, lumbar arteries; LCFA, lateral circumflex femoral arteries; LPIA, lateral posterior intercostal arteries; LSA, lateral sacral arteries; LTA, lateral thoracic artery; MCFA, medial circumflex femoral artery; SCIA, superficial circumflex iliac artery; SGA, superior gluteal artery; TCT, thyrocervical trunk; TDA, thoracodorsal artery. (*From* Geddes CR, Tang M, Yang D, et al. In: Blondeel PN, Morris SF, Hallock GG, et al, editors. Perforator flaps, anatomy, technique and clinical applications. St Louis (MO): Quality Medical Publishing; 2006. Fig. 18–3, p. 365, Chapter 18; with permission.)

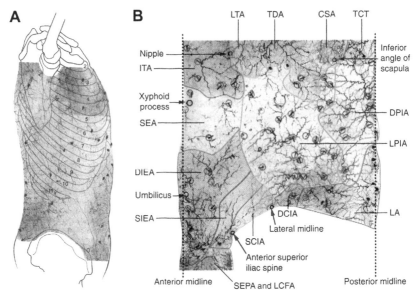

Fig. 17. (*A*) Angiogram of the integument of the lateral trunk. (*B*) Colored vascular territories of the various source vessels are shown. CSA, circumflex scapular artery; DCIA, deep circumflex iliac artery; DIEA, deep inferior epigastric artery; DPIA, dorsal posterior intercostal arteries; EPA, external pudendal artery; ILA, iliolumbar artery; ITA, internal thoracic artery; LA, lumbar arteries; LCFA, lateral circumflex femoral arteries; LPIA, lateral posterior intercostal arteries; LTA, lateral thoracic artery; SCIA, superficial circumflex iliac artery; SEA, superior epigastric artery; SEPA, superior external pudendal artery; SGA, superior gluteal artery; SIEA, superficial inferior epigastric artery; TCT, thyrocervical trunk; TDA, thoracodorsal artery. (*From* Geddes CR, Tang M, Yang D, et al. In: Blondeel PN, Morris SF, Hallock GG, et al, editors. Perforator flaps, anatomy, technique and clinical applications. St Louis (MO): Quality Medical Publishing; 2006. Fig. 18–3, p. 365, Chapter 18; with permission.)

axis, the descending aorta, and the external iliac arteries. Superiorly, branches from the subclavian/axillary axis, including the internal and lateral thoracic, thyrocervical, thoracoacromial, and subscapular arteries, supply the chest, axilla, and part of the upper back. Posteriorly, the descending thoracic and abdominal aorta gives off the segmental posterior intercostal, subcostal, and lumbar arteries. Inferiorly, perforators from the epigastric and circumflex iliac branches of the external iliac and common femoral arteries supply the lower abdominal region. The primary vascular supply to the external genitalia and perineum is via perforators from the internal and external pudendal, perineal, and inferior rectal arteries.

The integument of the trunk covers approximately 30% of the surface area of the body. An average of 122 perforators from 16 vascular territories supplies the integument. The average diameter and area supplied by a single perforator from the trunk region are approximately 0.7 mm and 40 cm^2, respectively.[12] The commonly harvested perforator flaps include the deep inferior epigastric flap (detailed in Dr Lipa's article on perforator flaps for breast reconstruction) and the thoracodorsal artery perforator flap (covered in Dr Hamdi's article on perforator flaps in the trunk).

CUTANEOUS VASCULATURE OF THE LOWER EXTREMITY

The lower extremity is the largest donor site in the body for perforator flap harvest. The iliac arterial system is the main arterial supply of the lower extremity. The superior and inferior gluteal arteries are the principal supply of the integument of the gluteal region. The branches of the superficial and profunda femoral arteries supply the thigh. Just proximal to the knee, the femoral artery passes to the posterior aspect of the thigh. As the vessel enters the popliteal fossa, it becomes the popliteal artery and continues to supply the integument of the knee. The popliteal artery terminates in the upper part of the leg by dividing into anterior and posterior tibial arteries. These vessels and their branches, including the peroneal artery, supply the integument of the leg. At the ankle, the anterior tibial artery becomes the dorsalis pedis artery which, along with the terminal branches of the posterior tibial and peroneal arteries, supplies the ankle and foot. The lower extremity, particularly the thigh, appears to have the greatest potential for harvesting new or modified perforator flaps.

An average of 93 perforators from 21 vascular territories supply the integument of the lower extremity (**Fig. 18**). The average diameter and area supplied by a single perforator is approximately 0.7 mm and 47 cm², respectively.[13] Many of the cutaneous perforators in the lower extremity, particularly in the thigh, are suitable as donor vessels for pedicled or free perforator flap harvest. In the thigh, there are a large number of large caliber perforators with long pedicle length. The anterolateral thigh flap, based on the descending branch of the lateral circumflex femoral artery, has become one of the most popular flaps and is known for its versatility (covered in detail in the article by Dr Neligan on the anterolateral thigh flap). Detailed vascular

anatomy of the buttock (**Fig. 19**), the thigh (**Fig. 20**), and the lower leg (**Fig. 21**) are shown.

The concept of free-style free flaps, coined by Wei and Mardini,[17] refers to the flexible surgical plan of harvest of the most suitable flap vessel for a specific flap. The concept was first applied mostly to the harvest of flaps in the thigh region because the region has a large number of suitable perforators. There are approximately 400 perforators in the body so there is a wide choice of donor sites for free-style perforator flap harvest.

The harvest of perforator flaps based on the medial circumflex femoral, posterior tibial,

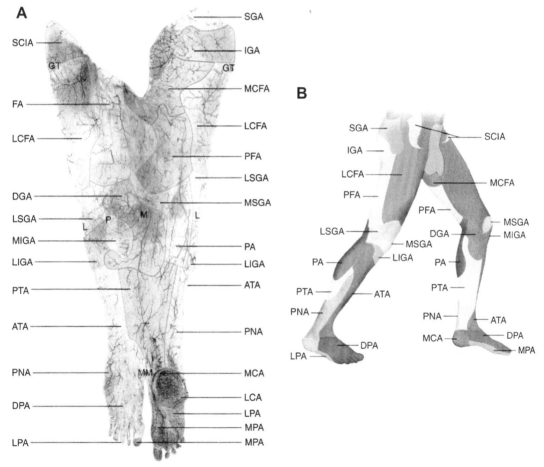

Fig. 18. Integument of the lower extremity. (*A*) Angiogram of the lower extremity of a human cadaver. (*B*) The vascular territories of the lower extremity. ATA, anterior tibial artery; DGA, descending geniculate artery; DPA, dorsalis pedis artery; FA, femoral artery; GT, greater trochanter; IGA, inferior gluteal artery; L, lateral epicondyle; LCA, lateral calcaneal artery; LCFA, lateral circumflex femoral artery; LIGA, lateral inferior genicular artery; LPA, lateral plantar artery; LSGA, lateral superior genicular artery; M, medial epicondyle; MCA, medial calcaneal artery; MCFA, medial circumflex femoral artery; MIGA, medial inferior genicular artery; MM, medial malleolus; MPA, medial plantar artery; MSGA, medial superior genicular artery; P, patella; PA, popliteal artery; PFA, profunda femoris artery; PNA, peroneal artery; PRA, posterior tibial artery; SCIA, superficial circumflex iliac artery; SGA, superior gluteal artery. (*From* Geddes CR, Tang M, Yang D, et al. In: Blondeel PN, Morris SF, Hallock GG, et al, editors. Perforator flaps, anatomy, technique and clinical applications. St Louis (MO): Quality Medical Publishing; 2006. Fig. 30–1, p. 544, Chapter 30; with permission.)

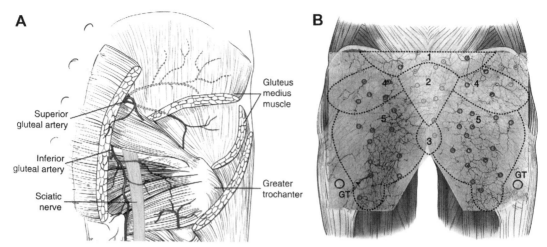

Fig. 19. (*A*) Vascular anatomy of the buttock. (*B*) Angiogram of the buttock showing musculocutaneous (*blue circles*) and septocutaneous (*red circles*) perforators. Perforators are from: 1, dorsal cutaneous branches of the lumbar artery; 2, lateral sacral artery; 3, internal pudendal; 4, superior gluteal artery; 5, inferior pudendal artery. GT, greater trochanter. (*From* Geddes CR, Tang M, Yang D, et al. In: Blondeel PN, Morris SF, Hallock GG, et al, editors. Perforator flaps, anatomy, technique and clinical applications. St Louis (MO): Quality Medical Publishing; 2006. Fig. 30–1, p. 544, Chapter 30; with permission.)

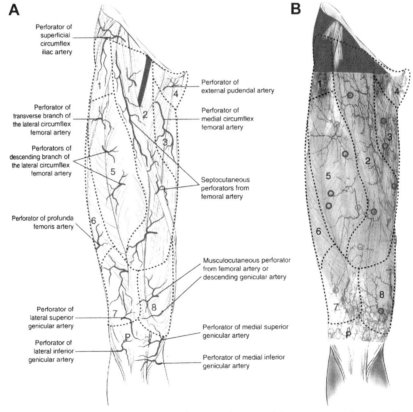

Fig. 20. Anterior thigh perforators. (*A*) Diagram of the perforators. (*B*) Angiogram showing the distribution of perforators in the thigh in a human cadaver. The red circles are musculocutaneous perforators and the blue circles are septocutaneous perforators. The anatomic territories shown are: 1, descending branch of the superficial circumflex iliac artery; 2, femoral artery; 3, medial circumflex femoral artery; 4, superficial external pudendal artery; 5, lateral circumflex femoral artery; 6, profunda femoris artery; 7, lateral superior genicular artery; 8, medial superior genicular artery. P, patella. (*From* Geddes CR, Tang M, Yang D, et al. In: Blondeel PN, Morris SF, Hallock GG, et al, editors. Perforator flaps, anatomy, technique and clinical applications. St Louis (MO): Quality Medical Publishing; 2006. Fig. 30–1, p. 544, Chapter 30; with permission.)

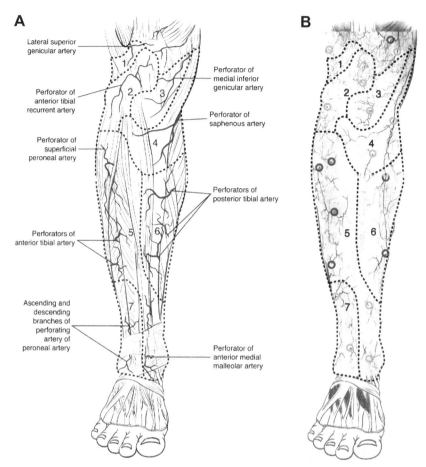

Fig. 21. Anterior lower leg perforators. (*A*) Diagram of the perforators. (*B*) Angiogram showing the distribution of perforators in the lower leg in a human cadaver. The red circles are musculocutaneous perforators and the blue circles are septocutaneous perforators. The anatomic territories shown are: 1, lateral inferior genicular artery; 2, anterior tibial recurrent branch of the anterior tibial artery; 3, medial inferior genicular artery; 4, descending genicular artery; 5, anterior tibial artery; 6, posterior tibial artery; 7, peroneal artery. (*From* Geddes CR, Tang M, Yang D, et al. In: Blondeel PN, Morris SF, Hallock GG, et al, editors. Perforator flaps, anatomy, technique and clinical applications. St Louis (MO): Quality Medical Publishing; 2006. Fig. 30–1, p. 544, Chapter 30; with permission.)

peroneal, and posterior tibial arteries has completely changed the pattern of flap use in lower-extremity reconstruction. In particular, propeller flaps have become an important tool in lower-limb reconstruction (Dr Teo covers this in detail in the article on propeller flaps elsewhere in this issue.) The series of perforators from the lower-leg vessels, the anterior tibial, the posterior tibial, and the peroneal are useful for lower-leg reconstruction (see **Fig. 21**).

PERFORATOR FLAP NOMENCLATURE

As the literature becomes increasingly filled with references to perforator flaps, the terminology used to describe novel flap designs can become confusing and difficult to interpret. In an effort to simplify the terminology, the authors introduced a nomenclature for perforator flaps that can be applied to all flaps.[18] This nomenclature became known as the Canadian classification. Basically, all flaps can be defined by the source vessel on which the flap is based. Hence, for a deep inferior epigastric artery flap, the flap would be known as a deep inferior epigastric perforator (DIEAP) flap. If there were different muscles that a musculocutaneous perforator could pass through, such as in the anterolateral thigh flap, this can be clarified with a suffix. For example, a flap based on a perforator from the descending branch of the lateral circumflex femoral artery passing through vastus lateralis would be a LCFAP-vl. Although no terminology or nomenclature system is perfect, the description of the main source vessel of a flap will clarify this evolving field of reconstructive surgery.

SUMMARY

Manchot, Salmon, and Taylor, among other anatomists, have provided contemporary surgeons with a vast amount of information to use in the daily search for ideal soft tissue cover. With more than 400 perforators to choose from, the challenge is to select the best perforator flap for each wound. An awareness of the anatomic details contained in this article will help surgeons to make the right choices.

REFERENCES

1. Taylor GI, Ives A, Dhar S. Vascular territories. In: Mathes S, editor. Plastic surgery. 3rd edition. Philadelphia: Elsevier; 2006.
2. Manchot C. The cutaneous arteries of the human body. Ristic J, Morain WD, trans, New York: Springer-Verlag; 1983.
3. Salmon M. Arteres de la Peau. Paris: Masson; 1936.
4. Taylor GI, Palmer JH. The vascular territories (angiosomes) of the body: Experimental study and clinical applications. Br J Plast Surg 1987;40:113–41.
5. Tang M, Yin Z, Morris SF. A pilot study on three-dimensional visualization of perforator flaps by using angiography in cadavers. Plast Reconstr Surg 2008; 122(2):429–37.
6. Tang M, Mao Y, Almutairi K, et al. Three-dimensional analysis of perforators of the posterior leg. Plast Reconstr Surg 2009;123(6):1729–38.
7. Tang, M, Morris, SF. Three-dimensional angiography of the deep circumflex iliac artery osteocutaneous perforator flap. A cadaver study. Plast Reconstr Surgery, in press.
8. Rees MJ, Taylor GI. A simplified lead oxido cadaver injection technique. Plast Reconstr Surg 1986;77:141.
9. Crosthwaite GL, Taylor GI, Palmer JH. A new radio-opaque injection technique for tissue preservation. Br J Plast Surg 1987;40:497.
10. Yang D, Tang M, Geddes CR, et al. Anatomy of the integument of the head and neck. In: Blondeel P, Morris SF, Hallock GG, et al, editors. Perforator flaps: anatomy, technique and clinical applications. St Louis (MO): QMP; 2006. p. 133–60.
11. Thomas BP, Geddes CR, Tang M, et al. The vascular supply of the integument of the upper extremity. In: Blondeel P, Morris SF, Hallock GG, et al, editors. Perforator flaps: anatomy, technique and clinical applications. St Louis (MO): QMP; 2006. p. 129–246.
12. Geddes CR, Morris SF, Tang M, et al. Anatomy of the integument of the trunk. In: Blondeel P, Morris SF, Hallock GG, et al, editors. Perforator flaps: anatomy, technique and clinical applications. St Louis (MO): QMP; 2006. p. 359–84.
13. Geddes CR, Tang M, Yang D, et al. Anatomy of the integument of the lower extremity. In: Blondeel P, Morris SF, Hallock GG, et al, editors. Perforator flaps: anatomy, technique and clinical applications. St Louis (MO): QMP; 2006. p. 541–78.
14. Tang M, Geddes CR, Yang D, et al. Modified lead oxide-gelatin injection technique for vascular studies. Clin Anat 2002;1:73–8.
15. Bergeron L, Tang M, Morris SF. A review of vascular injection techniques for the study of perforator flaps. Plast Reconstr Surg 2006;117(6):2050–7.
16. Rozen WM, Ashtom MW, Le Roux CM, et al. The perforator angiosome: a new concept in the design of deep inferior epigastric artery perforator flaps for breast reconstruction. Microsurgery 2009;30(1): 1–7.
17. Wei FC, Mardini S. Free-style free flaps. Plast Reconstr Surg 2004;114:910–4.
18. Geddes CR, Morris SF, Neligan PC. Perforator flaps: evolution, classification and applications. Ann Plast Surg 2003;50:90–9.

Where do Perforator Flaps Fit in our Armamentarium?

Julian J. Pribaz, MD*, Rodney K. Chan, MD

KEYWORDS

- Perforator flaps • History • Muscle • Musculocutaneous
- Fasciocutaneous • Reconstruction

The reconstructive surgeon needs to be familiar with the full spectrum of reconstructive options, and select the method of reconstruction that will give the best aesthetic and functional outcome. Perforator flaps are the most recent, and without doubt the most exciting addition to our armamentarium as reconstructive surgeons. New flaps are being described with great rapidity, and it can be difficult to keep up with the pace of progress occurring in our specialty.

This fact is especially true for surgeons who have been in practice for several years and who have already incorporated into their practice the many innovations that preceded popularization of perforator flaps. While it is important to keep up to date and be progressive, it is also important not to give up the true and tried methods that have been successfully used for years, thus risking doing harm to patients by attempting newly described procedures without adequate preparation. One has to be aware that every new procedure has a learning curve, which can be steep. Perforator flaps certainly fall into this category for the novice who is not experienced in the relevant anatomy and the requisite fine dissections. Furthermore, it is important to realize that not all new procedures will stand the test of time. Although they may progress through a period of popularity initially, any increased complication rate may relegate them to the "list of procedures that I no longer do," a common list among some plastic surgeons.

As it turns out, many of the flaps that surgeons have used for years are in fact perforator flaps, although they have been known by another name. Without doubt, the recent emphasis on perforator flaps has enhanced our understanding of how flaps receive their blood supply. When it comes to raising flaps, it is the blood supply that is critical rather than the type of tissue in the flap. Thus, the change in nomenclature emphasizing the blood supply to the flap is a step forward. This advance is especially true for the musculocutaneous flaps, where the nutrient blood flow to the skin is dependent on perforating vessels and not the underlying muscle. There is no doubt that perforator flaps are here to stay and they have greatly increased the number of flap options for reconstruction. However, the extent to which the individual surgeon will incorporate newer perforator flaps into his or her "reconstructive ladder" or "elevator" will differ and continue to evolve. Ongoing debates and discussions on this exciting addition will be beneficial for our specialty.

Here the authors propose to briefly review the historical aspects of flap development and provide an overview of the senior author's (J.J.P.) personal experience with perforator flaps. Further, this expansive choice of flaps has led to a change in emphasis in our reconstructive efforts, with improved selection and refinements.

A HISTORICAL PERSPECTIVE

As already alluded to, the options available to the reconstructive surgeon have increased greatly over the last 40 years. It has been both exciting and a privilege to be a part of this process. It is

The authors receive no financial support for this work.
Division of Plastic Surgery, Brigham and Women's Hospital, 75 Francis Street, Boston, MA 02115, USA
* Corresponding author.
E-mail address: jpribaz@partners.org

Clin Plastic Surg 37 (2010) 571–579
doi:10.1016/j.cps.2010.06.007

hard to imagine what it was like to practice our specialty in the days of Sir Harold Gillies and other pioneers in the early part of the twentieth century, who were confronted with the daunting task of repairing terrible and devastating war injuries.[1] Although these early pioneers were innovative, patient, and persistent, they had very few choices to draw upon. Gillies recognized that "tissue transfer was a constant battle between blood supply and beauty," but it was the lack of detailed knowledge of the way skin obtains its blood supply that delayed advances at that time. Small defects were repaired with skin grafts or local random pedicle flaps, which were sometimes extended by applying the principles of delay. Other than the deltopectoral flap described by Bakamjian,[2] there were very few regional flaps. For larger defects, multistaged tube pedicle flaps, first described by Filatov[3] and popularized by Gillies and others, were used. This practice continued well into the 1960s.

The concept of axial flaps evolved in the 1970s, and a major discovery was the pedicle groin flap described by MacGregor and Jackson.[4,5] A new era began when it was realized that axial flaps could be detached and transferred as free flaps. It was the development of the practice of microsurgery by Buncke[6] and others that fueled the discovery of new flaps. The breakthrough occurred when the first cutaneous free flap was reported in Melbourne by Taylor and Daniel,[7] soon followed by O'Brien and Shanmugan[8] and several others. However, at that time there really were no other commonly known cutaneous flaps other than the groin flap, and the focus was on flap survival.

It became apparent that a more detailed anatomy of the vascular supply to the skin and its contents was required to not only increase the donor options, but to allow better flap selection and refinement. The outcome was a major renaissance in anatomic research. It was realized that in many regions of the body, the skin obtains its blood supply through the underlying muscles. This finding led to the discovery of many musculocutaneous flaps by Ger, Orticochea, McGraw, and others,[9–12] thus greatly expanding the repertoire of the reconstructive surgeon.

At the same time Ponten[13] observed that the inclusion of the deep fascia in extremity reconstruction led to hardier, more reliable flaps. These "super" flaps marked the beginning of fasciocutaneous flaps. As new muscle, musculocutaneous flaps, and fasciocutaneous flaps were being described, there was a real need to return to the cadaver laboratory to practice and perfect the harvest of these various flaps. Flap courses became common and an essential part of residency training. There followed an intense attempt to classify and categorize these newly described muscle and musculocutaneous flaps by Mathes and Nahai, and fasciocutaneous flaps by Cormack and Lamberty, among others.[14–17] The reconstructive ladder was rapidly lengthening, with more options available. The focus then changed to flap refinement.

The body of knowledge was further augmented by Taylor and Palmer,[18] who not only rediscovered the largely forgotten works of Manchot and Salmon,[19–22] but also performed their own extensive injection studies and cadaver dissections. These investigators further elucidated the arterial, venous, and lymphatic circulation to the skin and its contents, enabling Taylor to propose the "angiosome concept" of interconnecting vascularity of the skin, which greatly helped our understanding of how flaps survive.[23] The realization that the major source vessels supplied nutritional blood flow to all tissues to which they traversed, although obvious now, has not always been appreciated. These major vessels and their main named branches send other smaller branches to supply the surrounding muscles, bones, joints, and all connective tissue, and eventually the skin. It was discovered that in most locations there were set patterns in the way that skin obtained its blood flow: (1) via direct branches from source vessels that penetrated the fascia, (2) via vessels that first traversed muscle or passed through septa between the muscle groups, or occasionally (3) via vessels that first supply the bone, tendon, nerves, and so forth, giving rise to the concept of perforator flaps.[24] Koshima, a superb ultra-microsurgeon, is credited with the early work that led to the practical application of perforator flaps.[25,26]

Taylor's anatomic dissections identified almost 400 good-sized arterial perforators (at least 0.5 mm diameter), which each supplied a volume of skin, and therefore were capable of serving as pedicles for flaps and theoretically could be detached and transferred as free flaps[7]; this obviously greatly increases the number of flaps available for reconstruction,[27] and Wei and colleagues[28] coined the term "freestyle flaps" to describe the many potential flaps that could be raised on any of these yet unnamed perforating pedicles. However, as more flaps were being reported, it again became necessary to categorize and classify these new modifications. A shift in emphasis from naming flaps according to the body of tissue it contained to its source blood supply was a major step forward. This change in nomenclature led to a better understanding and reflected a more profound awareness of why some flaps were not always reliable. An example of this is the gracilis musculocutaneous flap, which traditionally is raised with a vertical skin island overlying the muscle. It is well known that the distal part of this vertical skin island is not reliable.

Yousif and colleagues[29] first pointed out that a transversely oriented skin island across the proximal third of the muscle is more reliable because it is richly supplied by the perforators from the medial circumflex femoral vessels that send branches through the muscle, as well as septal cutaneous perforators on either side of the muscle. Astute observations such as these help refine our reconstructive ladder.

With the potential for hundreds of new flaps, it became imperative to come to a consensus with naming and classification. An international meeting in Gent was helpful in developing the new nomenclature.[30,31] There have also been several proposals for flap classification. Nakajima and colleagues[32] have provided a very useful classification of the 6 different pathways through which blood flows from the source vessels to the skin. This classification has been further simplified according to the ease of pedicle dissection, as "direct perforators" from source vessel regardless of how it gets to the skin, and "indirect perforators" that are more difficult to dissect as these traverse the muscle first.[24]

GENERAL CONSIDERATIONS

It has been an exciting time to have been part of all these developments that have increased our knowledge base and greatly augmented and refined our arsenal of reconstructive options. Although some advocates of perforator flaps see this as a new field of reconstructive surgery, others, including the authors, see this more as a major refinement that has added some sophisticated subgroups to our reconstructive ladder.

The question then arises: how and when do we apply these principles to our practice? As in any surgical endeavor, reconstruction begins first by making an accurate diagnosis of the problem, visualizing what is missing, and then seeking the best way to achieve the optimal functional and aesthetic result, with the least donor site morbidity. Availability of perforator flaps has increased our choices greatly, often simplifying what has to be done.

There is a large array of reliable flaps of various sizes and compositions at our disposal that can be transferred as free flaps to reconstruct a distant defect. Further, having a better knowledge of the blood supply has enabled us to better tailor the flaps and refine the reconstructions. However, an even more beneficial and exciting development has been the possibility of using tissue close to or even adjacent to the defect as a local perforator flap. This technique not only provides a simpler and more expeditious repair, but arguably a superior aesthetic result because of better tissue match.

The increased availability of local flap options, a direct result of applied knowledge from perforator flap research, has enabled the reconstructive surgeon "to walk down the reconstructive ladder" to a simpler, local solution for a problem that in previous years had required a free flap.

Flap design according to the angiosome concept championed by Taylor generally works well for most truncal and extremity flaps, but there are some exceptions and regional differences where modifications are needed.[23] Taylor postulated that skin received its blood supply by a series of central, substantial perforating vascular pedicles, containing an artery and its venae comitantes. These perforating pedicles arborize and connect with other similar vascular territories via both true anastomotic vessels as well as reduced-caliber, choke vessels. In general, a flap can be safely raised with the next adjacent vascular territory, but not beyond that without prior delay. The delay process acts to open up the choke vessels between the vascular territories, so that a larger flap may be harvested.[18]

However, besides these perforating arteriovenous pedicles there are also separate, more superficial, longitudinally running venous and lymphatic systems, which are also important and need to be considered in flap design. Moreover in certain areas such as the central part of the face, there is a paucity of any substantial comitante veins. Instead there is a very fine syncytial venous plexus that nonetheless provides adequate venous drainage. Thus, in raising axial and perforator flaps in the central face, it is imperative to maintain some soft tissue surrounding the arterial inflow to provide venous drainage.[33–35] The lack of suitably sized veins accompanying the facial artery and its branches in this area has made replantation of amputated parts very difficult and unreliable. A similar situation exists in the distal limb and digits where the digital arteries have very small, rudimentary, and unusable venae comitantes, with the venous drainage being separate from the arterial inflow located on the dorsal aspect of the digit.

Elsewhere in the body, venous drainage of flaps occurs through the deep perforating comitante veins as well as by the superficial venous system. The contribution of venous drainage of these 2 systems can vary from patient to patient and from location to location. Even the very reliable and hardy radial forearm fasciocutaneous free flap not uncommonly requires an additional superficial venous anastomosis to adequately drain the flap.[36]

It has also been noted that in other areas, for example, in raising a deep inferior epigastric artery perforator (DIEAP) flap, if there is a large superficial inferior epigastric vein the possibility of venous congestion can be anticipated, especially if a large flap is raised.[37] Another interesting observation in certain areas, including the DIEAP vascular territory, is that often a hardy flap can be raised that extends well beyond 2 to 3 vascular territories. In this case, presumably there are large true anastomotic connections rather than reduced-caliber choke vessels. However, when a flap does extend beyond the next angiosome, it is not uncommon to encounter partial flap loss of the most distal part of the flap. This situation is usually caused by venous congestion, and may be remedied by providing additional venous drainage by either leaving an intact skin bridge at the base of the flap to allow for retrograde drainage by the superficial venous system or by performing an additional venous anastomosis of the superficial vein within the flap and at a distance from the perforating pedicle.[38]

It is clear that our understanding of the complexities of the blood supply, although greatly enhanced by all the research and experience with perforator flaps, is still incomplete and warrants further study.

CURRENT STATUS OF PERFORATOR FLAPS IN OUR RECONSTRUCTIVE ARMAMENTARIUM

As reconstructive surgeons we have all been beneficiaries of this extensive new body of knowledge that has emerged from perforator flap investigations. It has added understanding to what we are already doing and has also led to some modifications in existing techniques. One of the exciting aspects of plastic and reconstructive surgery is the constant changes, refinements, and modifications, adding to a growing list of "what we no longer do" due to the introduction of improved techniques to solve clinical problems.

The authors do not subscribe to the supposition by several zealots in the field that we have entered into a completely new era and subspecialty, where the answer to all problems is a perforator flap. Although embracing many of the newer concepts, the authors continue to value and use tried and proven older flaps and techniques in their practice algorithms. When there are multiple ways of solving a problem, it is understandable that there will be a variety of opinions and a healthy debate as to the merit of different techniques. Any new

concept or technique takes some time to become fully accepted by all and to eventually find its rightful place in a reconstructive armamentarium.

To help answer the question posed in the title of this article, namely, the current role of perforator flaps in our armamentarium, and the extent to which a significant change in practice paradigm has occurred, it is important to realize that generalization is not possible. It is fair to say that this will vary from region (or country) to region, from surgeon to surgeon, and also from one body part to the next. There are also economic and social factors that come into play in helping set the local norm of practice profiles, and thereby affect the hierarchy of choices a surgeon considers when selecting a procedure from the reconstructive ladder. Thus, the following represents the senior author's current practice and biases, which may be subject to change, and which may vary considerably with other opinions and practices. An in-depth discussion of the reconstructive modalities preferred in the different body regions is obviously beyond the scope of this article, and thus what follows is a much abbreviated summary of the current preferred reconstructive armamentarium.

HEAD AND NECK

Wherever possible, a local flap option that provides the best aesthetic and functional result is preferred. This option includes the use of local advancement, and rotation flaps of the cheek, though random at their distal parts, are nonetheless hardy and reliable, giving superior aesthetic results when compared with distant flaps.[34]

The rich blood supply by the facial artery and its branches centrally and other branches of the external and internal carotid tree provide a rich donor source for multiple pedicle perforator flaps.[34,35,39] These flaps include perforator-type flaps from the angular vessels (Island flaps, VY flaps) for nasal reconstruction,[40,41] facial artery musculomucosal flaps for intraoral and vermilion reconstruction,[33,42,43] median forehead flaps for nasal reconstruction, ascending helical free flaps for distal nasal reconstruction, and submental flaps for cutaneous and intraoral reconstructions.[44,45] The submental flaps can also help repair the beard area in males and can further be designed as a functional flap by including a segment of innervated underlying platysma muscle.[46]

Regional flaps, including temporoparietal fascial flaps, temporalis muscle flaps (often functional), pectoralis, trapezius, latissimus, and supraclavicular flaps, are also used.

With larger defects, free tissue transfers are required and a wide range of distant perforator flaps are commonly used, including the radial forearm flap, anterolateral thigh flap, and all the common osteocutaneous flaps when needed. With deeper and complex defects, muscle and musculocutaneous flaps are still very often used for the initial reconstruction. Subsequently, local flaps with better color and texture match may be used to enhance the external final appearance of the reconstruction.[34,35,47]

Also in my practice I use the techniques of flap prefabrication and prelamination in selected, complex reconstructions.[47] Prefabrication refers to creating an axial-like pedicle flap by prior implantation of a ligated vascular pedicle into a desired cutaneous area and then waiting approximately 2 months for neovascularization to occur before the flap is transferred. This process can be done at a distance to create thin flaps for reconstruction, although recently this has been replaced by the availability of thin perforator flaps. Alternatively, and perhaps even better still, the prefabrication process can occur locally where there is skin of better color and texture match for use in facial reconstruction.[48]

Prelamination, on the other hand, refers to creating flaps with multiple layers to reconstruct complex, central facial defects.[49] These flaps are created in preexisting vascular territories—most commonly in the radial forearm, and also locally in the submental region. After the various components have healed and the multilayered flap created, it is transferred to the face to repair a complex, central defect. However, secondary revisions that use local flaps are routinely performed to enhance the final aesthetic result.[50–53]

UPPER EXTREMITY

The upper extremity has major source arteries that traverse the limb and give multiple musculocutaneous and septocutaneous perforators to the skin. There exist also rich anastomotic networks around the joints from which multiple fasciocutaneous flaps arise. Because of these rich anastomotic networks, it is possible to raise direct cutaneous flaps that are both proximally and distally based. Distally based flaps from source vessels (eg, radial forearm) will have a retrograde blood flow, but are generally very reliable. Perforator flaps arising from main source vessels (eg, dorsal ulna branch) may be proximally or distally based but still have an orthograde flow, in keeping with Taylor's angiosome concept. A full spectrum of local and regional flaps is commonly used, including the many different types of small flaps used in hand and digital reconstruction, which are not listed here. It should be remembered that

even in patients with burns that have previously been grafted, it is still possible to raise many flaps because the perforators remain intact deep to the fascia and can support a mature skin-grafted fascial flap.[54,55]

Major trauma and tissue loss require distant flaps and this generally involves free tissue transfers, with a preference for fasciocutaneous flaps rather than skin-grafted muscle flaps.[56] These flaps may require secondary debulking, but I believe a better aesthetic result is achieved. It is also easier to perform secondary reconstructive procedures on tendons and bones when operating through a skin flap rather than skin-grafted muscle. The use of flap material from the foot (toes, joints, and so forth) is commonly used as needed. The pedicled groin flap is still used in my practice, especially for patients with extensive soft-tissue injuries that will require a major subsequent microsurgical procedure such as a toe transfer. The groin flap can be designed not only to provide an abundance of cutaneous coverage but also to spare recipient vessels for later microsurgery. In devastating injuries, the use of "spare parts" surgery with rearrangement of injured parts dissected on their vascular pedicles is also worth considering in our reconstructive armamentarium.[57]

BREAST RECONSTRUCTION

There is no doubt that breast reconstruction with autogenous tissue gives superior results. The impact of perforator flaps in breast reconstruction has been great, but in no other area of reconstruction is there more controversy and debate as to the relative merits of different types of autogenous reconstruction, especially between advocates of free DIEAP flaps and pedicle transverse rectus abdominis myocutaneous (TRAM) flaps. In experienced hands, excellent results can be obtained by both free-tissue flap and pedicle flap reconstructions. Intuitively there should be less donor site morbidity with perforator-type flaps, as long as there is minimal muscle and nerve damage during flap harvest; however, there are no good prospective studies to date that convincingly support one method over the other.

There are major geographic differences with respect to the preferred method of breast reconstruction. Most plastic surgeons in Europe and Asia perform free perforator flap methods of reconstruction almost exclusively, whereas in the United States the pedicle TRAM flap is still the most popular method for autogenous reconstruction. The reason for these geographic differences are multifactorial and are related to training, as well as economic factors and a desire to super-specialize and restrict clinical practice to breast surgery.

In many European countries, trainees are not taught to do pedicle TRAM flaps, but instead are mainly schooled in performing perforator flaps. Pedicle TRAM flaps are then often relegated to nonplastic surgeons, with inferior results and higher complication rates. Such is not the case in the United States. When properly done, I believe that both methods of reconstruction can give excellent results with comparable donor site morbidity.

I believe that there are also economic factors that affect the method of reconstruction selected from our reconstructive armamentarium. In most states, perforator flaps that take longer to perform are currently and rightly better reimbursed than pedicle TRAM flaps. However, one does wonder what would happen to the flap selection process should changes occur to our health care policy and reimbursement. Furthermore, the increased complexity and time commitment of perforator flap breast reconstruction, coupled with the increasing demand for mastectomy and reconstruction, has literally swamped many of these surgeons thus limiting their reconstructive practices to breast exclusively. I believe that this latter reason is also a significant factor in determining the extent to which a surgeon elects to selectively use the free perforator method of breast reconstruction. In my practice, I perform mainly pedicle TRAM flaps for breast reconstruction, but occasionally I also use free TRAMs, DIEAP flaps, and superior gluteal artery perforator flaps, as well as latissimus dorsi flaps.

For a partial breast reconstruction, I commonly use perforator flaps based on the thoracodorsal system as pedicle flaps to reconstruct these defects.

TRUNK AND CHEST WALL

The defects involving the anterior chest wall are often complex, deep, and irregular. These defects are often infected with exposed bone and hardware. In these situations, the use of muscle and musculocutaneous flaps is generally preferred over the use of perforator flaps. For sternal wounds and chest wall defects, the commonly used flaps include the pectoralis major flap, TRAM flap, latissimus dorsi flap (if still available and not rendered unusable due to transection by the thoracic surgeons) and, occasionally, a pedicled omental flap. Often a combination of these flaps, including a free flap option, is required to adequately repair large complex defects.

On the posterior aspect of the trunk, the latissimus dorsi flap and trapezius myocutaneous flaps are very commonly used, especially for deep and complex defects. For spinal defects with exposed hardware and markedly irregular defects, often small local paraspinal muscle flaps are used to obliterate the dead space and are supplemented with larger local musculocutaneous and fasciocutaneous flaps for coverage.

In the lower back where the reach of muscle and musculocutaneous flaps is limited, perforator flaps from either the lumbar vessels or from the superior gluteal vessels may be used. For larger defects, free tissue transfers are generally required.

BUTTOCK REGION

The need for flap reconstruction in this region is mainly for reconstruction of defects following pressure sore debridement. Such defects typically occur in patients who are paraplegic or quadriplegic but may occasionally occur also in patients who are ambulatory, and muscle-sparing techniques are required. The perforators to the skin in this region are mostly all musculocutaneous, and traditionally muscle and musculocutaneous flaps have been used. These are very suitable flaps for repairing deep and complex wounds, where the muscle can conform and fill the irregularly shaped wound. However, because of the thick subcutaneous layer in this region, pedicled perforator flaps with a generous arc of rotation may also be used to adequately fill even deep wounds. Furthermore, the use of perforator flaps preserves the underlying muscle, providing a "lifeboat" for any recurrent problems. Thus in this region there is an increasing popularity of perforator-type flaps, and most flaps are based on the perforators from the superior and inferior gluteal vessels. Perforator flaps are also commonly used from the upper thigh region, especially for ischial and trochanteric pressure sores.

PERINEAL AND PELVIC RECONSTRUCTION

This region commonly presents the reconstructive surgeon with major extirpative defects requiring bulky flap reconstruction, and for this reason musculocutaneous flaps, especially from the abdomen, such as the vertical rectus abdominis musculocutaneous flap and the TRAM flap, are commonly used. In addition, musculocutaneous and perforator flaps from the upper medial thigh are also commonly used for perineal defects. Less often, there may be a need for a thinner flap, such as for penile, scrotal, or even vaginal reconstruction. In these situations, a perforator-type flap such as from the DIEAP system and other flaps including free flaps may be used.

LOWER EXTREMITY

Like the upper extremity, the lower extremity has deep source arteries that traverse the limb with multiple perforators passing through the muscles of the thigh and calf as well as septal perforators passing around the muscles. Around the hip, knee, ankle joints, and foot there is a rich anastomotic network, and fasciocutaneous perforator flaps are commonly used. The thigh has become the most frequently used donor site for distant free flaps, especially flaps arising from the descending branch of the lateral femoral circumflex vascular pedicle. This area is a prime donor site about which the authors reported their early experience long before this flap became popular in the United States.[58,59] The authors found, as others have found since, that two-thirds of the perforators that come from the source vessels are musculocutaneous and one-third septocutaneous. The descending lateral femoral circumflex pedicle, which is long and robust, has also been commonly used as the pedicle for flap prefabrication.[50–53]

In the lower extremity, the use of perforator flaps has greatly changed our practice paradigm and has led to simpler methods of reconstruction, especially in the distal third of the leg for which the classic teaching has been that free flaps are required.[60] The use of perforator flaps, especially from the peroneal system, including the reverse sural flap, and other flaps based on vessels that run with nerves in this area such as the saphenous flap, the dorsalis pedis myofascial flap, and the medial plantar fasciocutaneous flaps are often used for reconstructing difficult areas in this region.[61–64] As mentioned earlier, where longer flaps are required it has been found safer to include a skin bridge at the base of the flap to assist with venous drainage.

SUMMARY

The use of perforator flaps is a new and exciting paradigm in reconstructive surgery. Some of these flaps are actually not new but are in fact older flaps now known to be based on a perforating vessel. Investigations in this area will no doubt result in expansive perforator flap options. More importantly, it will hopefully shed more light on the intricacies of flap vascularity.

A large array of reliable perforator flaps of various sizes and compositions that can be transferred as free flaps is reviewed here. However, the possibility of using tissue adjacent to the defect as a local perforator flap can provide a simpler and more expeditious repair.

The extent to which each individual surgeon will incorporate these newly described flaps into his or her reconstructive repertoire will depend on many factors, which the authors have tried to summarize in this article.

REFERENCES

1. Gillies HD. Plastic surgery of facial burns. Surg Gynaecol Obstet 1920;30:121–34.
2. Bakamjian VY. A two-stage method for pharyngoesophageal reconstruction with a primary pectoral skin flap. Plast Reconstr Surg 1965;36:173–84.
3. Filatov VP. Plastic procedure using a round pedicle. Vestn Oftalmol 1917;34:149 [in Russian].
4. McGregor IA, Jackson IT. The groin flap. Br J Plast Surg 1972;25(1):3–16.
5. McGregor IA, Morgan O. Axial and random pattern flaps. Br J Plast Surg 1973;26(3):202–13.
6. Buncke H. Recent advances in microsurgery. Calif Med 1970;113(5):66–7.
7. Taylor GI, Daniel RK. The free flap: composite tissue transfer by vascular anastomosis. Aust N Z J Surg 1973;43(1):1–3.
8. O'Brien BM, Shanmugan N. Experimental transfer of composite free flaps with microvascular anastomoses. Aust N Z J Surg 1973;43(3):285–8.
9. Ger R. The technique of muscle transposition in the operative treatment of traumatic and ulcerative lesions of the leg. J Trauma 1971;11(6):502–10.
10. Orticochea M. The musculocutaneous flap method as a substitute for the method of delayed transfer. Report on a discovery. Acta Chir Plast 1983;25(1):6–13.
11. McCraw JB, Dibbell DG. Experimental definition of independent myocutaneous vascular territories. Plast Reconstr Surg 1977;60(2):212–20.
12. McCraw JB, Dibbell DG, Carraway JH. Clinical definition of independent myocutaneous vascular territories. Plast Reconstr Surg 1977;60(3):341–52.
13. Ponten B. The fasciocutaneous flap: its use in soft tissue defects of the lower leg. Br J Plast Surg 1981;34(2):215–20.
14. Mathes SJ, Nahai F. Classification of the vascular anatomy of muscles: experimental and clinical correlation. Plast Reconstr Surg 1981;67(2):177–87.
15. Cormack G, Lamberty B. The arterial anatomy of skin flaps. Edinburgh (UK): Churchill Livingstone; 1986.
16. Cormack G, Lamberty B. The anatomical basic for fasciocutaneous flaps. Cambridge (MA): Blackwell Scientific Publications; 1992.
17. Cormack G, Lamberty B. The fasciocutaneous system of vessels. Arterial anatomy of skin flaps. Edinburgh (UK): Churchill Livingstone; 1994. p. 105–29.
18. Taylor GI, Palmer JH. The vascular territories (angiosomes) of the body: experimental study and clinical applications. Br J Plast Surg 1987;40(2):113–41.
19. Manchot C. Die hautarterien de menschlichen korpers. Leipzig (Germany): FCW Vogel; 1889.
20. Manchot C. The cutaneous arteries of the human body. New York: Springer-Verlag; 1982.
21. Salmon M. Arteres de la peau. Paris (France): Masson; 1936.

22. Salmon M, Taylor G, Tempest M. Arteries of the skin. London: Churchill-Livingstone; 1988.

23. Taylor GI. The angiosomes of the body and their supply to perforator flaps. Clin Plast Surg 2003; 30(3):331–42, v.

24. Hallock GG. Direct and indirect perforator flaps: the history and the controversy. Plast Reconstr Surg 2003;111(2):855–65 [quiz: 866].

25. Koshima I, Soeda S. Inferior epigastric artery skin flaps without rectus abdominis muscle. Br J Plast Surg 1989;42(6):645–8.

26. Koshima I, Moriguchi T, Fukuda H, et al. Free, thinned, paraumbilical perforator-based flaps. J Reconstr Microsurg 1991;7(4):313–6.

27. Mardini S, Tsai FC, Wei FC. The thigh as a model for free style free flaps. Clin Plast Surg 2003;30(3):473–80.

28. Wei FC, Jain V, Suominen S, et al. Confusion among perforator flaps: what is a true perforator flap? Plast Reconstr Surg 2001;107(3):874–6.

29. Yousif NJ, Matloub HS, Kolachalam R, et al. The transverse gracilis musculocutaneous flap. Ann Plast Surg 1992;29(6):482–90.

30. Blondeel PN, Van Landuyt KH, Monstrey SJ, et al. The "Gent" consensus on perforator flap terminology: preliminary definitions. Plast Reconstr Surg 2003;112(5):1378–83 [quiz: 1383, 1516; discussion: 1384–7].

31. Taylor G. The "Gent" consensus on perforator flap terminology: preliminary definitions. Plast Reconstr Surg 2003;112(5):1384–7 [discussion].

32. Nakajima H, Fujino T, Adachi S. A new concept of vascular supply to the skin and classification of skin flaps according to their vascularization. Ann Plast Surg 1986;16(1):1–19.

33. Pribaz J, Stephens W, Crespo L, et al. A new intraoral flap: facial artery musculomucosal (FAMM) flap. Plast Reconstr Surg 1992;90(3):421–9.

34. Chun Y, Pribaz J. Soft tissue reconstruction in face and neck. In: Butler C, editor. Head and neck surgery. Oxford: Saunders Elsevier; 2009. p. 1–38.

35. Chun Y, Pribaz J. Facial soft tissue reconstruction. In: Nelligan P, Wei FC, editors. Microsurgical reconstruction of the head and neck. St Louis (MO): Quality Medical Publishing, Inc.; 2009. p. 449–93.

36. Liu Y, Jiang X, Huang J, et al. Reliability of the superficial venous drainage of the radial forearm free flaps in oral and maxillofacial reconstruction. Microsurgery 2008;28(4):243–7.

37. Villafane O, Gahankari D, Webster M. Superficial inferior epigastric vein (SIEV): 'lifeboat' for DIEP/TRAM flaps. Br J Plast Surg 1999;52(7):599.

38. Drever JM, Hodson-Walker NJ. Immediate breast reconstruction after mastectomy using a rectus abdominal myodermal flap without an implant. Can J Surg 1982;25(4):429–31.

39. Parrett BM, Pribaz JJ. An algorithm for treatment of nasal defects. Clin Plast Surg 2009;36(3):407–20.

40. Guo L, Pribaz JR, Pribaz JJ. Nasal reconstruction with local flaps: a simple algorithm for management of small defects. Plast Reconstr Surg 2008;122(5): 130e–9e.

41. Hofer SO, Posch NA, Smit X. The facial artery perforator flap for reconstruction of perioral defects. Plast Reconstr Surg 2005;115(4):996–1003 [discussion: 1004–5].

42. Pribaz JJ, Meara JG, Wright S, et al. Lip and vermilion reconstruction with the facial artery musculomucosal flap. Plast Reconstr Surg 2000;105(3):864–72.

43. Warren S, Pribaz J. Facial artery musculomucosal flap. In: Blondeel P, Hallock GG, Morris S, et al, editors. Perforator flaps: anatomy, technique and clinical applications. St Louis (MO): Quality Medical Publishing, Inc.; 2006. p. 181–97.

44. Pribaz JJ, Falco N. Nasal reconstruction with auricular microvascular transplant. Ann Plast Surg 1993; 31(4):289–97.

45. Taghinia AH, Movassaghi K, Wang AX, et al. Reconstruction of the upper aerodigestive tract with the submental artery flap. Plast Reconstr Surg 2009; 123(2):562–70.

46. Fine NA, Pribaz JJ, Orgill DP. Use of the innervated platysma flap in facial reanimation. Ann Plast Surg 1995;34(3):326–30 [discussion: 330–1].

47. Pribaz JJ, Fine NA. Prelamination: defining the prefabricated flap—a case report and review. Microsurgery 1994;15(9):618–23.

48. Pribaz JJ, Fine N, Orgill DP. Flap prefabrication in the head and neck: a 10-year experience. Plast Reconstr Surg 1999;103(3):808–20.

49. Pribaz JJ, Weiss DD, Mulliken JB, et al. Prelaminated free flap reconstruction of complex central facial defects. Plast Reconstr Surg 1999;104(2): 357–65 [discussion: 366–7].

50. Pribaz JJ, Fine NA. Prefabricated and prelaminated flaps for head and neck reconstruction. Clin Plast Surg 2001;28(2):261–72, vii.

51. Pribaz J, Guo L. Flap prefabrication and prelamination in head and neck reconstruction. Semin Plast Surg 2003;17(4):351–62 flaps in head and neck reconstruction, Part 2.

52. Parrett BM, Pribaz J. Prefabricated and prelaminated flaps. In: Nelligan P, Wei FC, editors. Microsurgical reconstruction of the head and neck. St Louis (MO): Quality Medical Publishing, Inc.; 2009. p. 845–60.

53. Mathy JA, Pribaz JJ. Prefabrication and prelamination applications in current aesthetic facial reconstruction. Clin Plast Surg 2009;36(3):493–505.

54. Pribaz JJ, Pelham FR. Use of previously burned skin in local fasciocutaneous flaps for upper extremity reconstruction. Ann Plast Surg 1994;33(3):272–80.

55. Chan R, Pribaz J. Use of previously burned skin flaps. In: Hyakusoka H, Ogawa R, editors. Atlas of burn reconstruction. Verlag Berlin: Springer; 2010. p. 330–7.

56. Orgill DP, Pribaz JJ, Morris DJ. Local fasciocutaneous flaps for olecranon coverage. Ann Plast Surg 1994;32(1):27–31.

57. Ganchi P, Pribaz J. Spare parts in upper extremity reconstruction. In: Weinzweig N, Weinzweig J, editors. The mutilated hand. Philadelphia: Elsevier Mosby; 2005. p. 441–60.

58. Pribaz JJ, Orgill DP, Epstein MD, et al. Anterolateral thigh free flap. Ann Plast Surg 1995;34(6):585–92.

59. Pribaz J, Mankani M. Anterolateral thigh flap. In: Russell R, editor. Flaps. St Louis: Mosby; 1999.

60. Parrott DM, Matros E, Pribaz JJ, et al. Lower extremity trauma: trends in the management of soft-tissue reconstruction of open tibia-fibula fractures. Plast Reconstr Surg 2006;117(4):1315–22 [discussion: 1323–4].

61. Orgill DP, Pribaz JJ. Reverse peroneal flaps: two surgical approaches. Ann Plast Surg 1994;33(1): 17–22.

62. Parrett BM, Pribaz JJ, Matros E, et al. Risk analysis for the reverse sural fasciocutaneous flap in distal leg reconstruction. Plast Reconstr Surg 2009; 123(5):1499–504.

63. Gibstein LA, Abramson DL, Sampson CE, et al. Musculofascial flaps based on the dorsalis pedis vascular pedicle for coverage of the foot and ankle. Ann Plast Surg 1996;37(2):152–7.

64. Masquelet AC, Romana MC, Wolf G. Skin island flaps supplied by the vascular axis of the sensitive superficial nerves: anatomic study and clinical experience in the leg. Plast Reconstr Surg 1992;89(6): 1115–21.

Preoperative Imaging Techniques for Perforator Selection in Abdomen-Based Microsurgical Breast Reconstruction

David W. Mathes, MD*,
Peter C. Neligan, MB, BCh, FRCS(I), FRCS(C), FACS

KEYWORDS

- Breast reconstruction • Perforator-based flap
- Postoperative imaging • Microsurgery

The clinical application of perforator-based flaps for microsurgical breast reconstruction has increased exponentially over the past 10 years.[1,2] The benefits of the procedure are thought to be that it produces less postoperative pain, lowers abdominal morbidity, and allows for better preservation of muscles at the donor site compared with conventional musculocutaneous flaps such as the transverse rectus abdominus myocutaneous (TRAM).[3–5] The disadvantages of perforator flaps are that they are more difficult to harvest, which can result in a longer operative time and higher costs. Furthermore, some still question the wisdom of basing large flaps on a single perforator and emphasize the increased rate of fat necrosis.[6]

The vascular anatomy of the deep inferior epigastric artery and its perforating branches in the abdominal wall varies greatly not only among individuals but also from one side of the abdomen to the other.[7] Perforator location, number, caliber, and the intramuscular trajectory of the branches all impact the design and harvest of the flap. The creation of a presurgical map of the vessels on the abdomen can facilitate surgical planning and could decrease operating room time, reduce intraoperative complications, and lead to improve outcomes.

This article reviews the available techniques for preoperative planning with the currently available imaging modalities: hand-held Doppler, color Doppler (duplex) ultrasound, CT angiography (CTA), and MR angiography (MRA).

DOPPLER ULTRASOUND

One of the most inexpensive and common techniques for locating perforators is the use of the unidirectional Doppler probe. The Doppler probe can be used by the surgeon in both the pre- and postoperative settings and a comparison made between pre- and postoperative signals.[8] The hand-held Doppler is available in all surgical operating suites and can be used to mark the relative location of perforators.[9] The downside of this device is that it may be too highly sensitive, and thereby often locates not only clinically significant perforators but also very small perforators that are insufficient to support the flap. This lack of specificity has been well documented in its use for locating perforators in the anterior lateral thigh flap.[10] Because of this lack of specificity,

Division of Plastic and Reconstructive Surgery, Department of Surgery, University of Washington School of Medicine, 1959 NE Pacific, Box 35640, Seattle, WA 98195, USA
* Corresponding author. Division of Plastic Surgery, Department of Surgery, University of Washington, Box 356410, Seattle, WA 98195-6410.
E-mail address: dwmathes@u.washington.edu

Clin Plastic Surg 37 (2010) 581–591
doi:10.1016/j.cps.2010.06.011

use of the hand-held Doppler alone has not been considered reliable for perforator mapping; it does not achieve the sensitivity and breadth of information available with the other imaging technologies. In addition, because of the significant time, low accuracy, and high interobserver variability associated with perforator mapping, unidirectional Doppler is not currently embraced as a suitable preoperative imaging modality. It remains a useful tool for intraoperative evaluation to document and follow the flow of a chosen perforator during dissection.

COLOR DUPLEX ULTRASOUND

Unlike the hand-held Doppler, which can only note the location of a perforator, color duplex ultrasound can provide information on both the perforator diameter and flow velocity (**Fig. 1**). After examination with color duplex ultrasound, a perforator map can be generated of the number and anatomic position of all perforators in relation to the abdominal skin. In addition, the examination can provide information on vessel damage caused by atherosclerosis, previous surgery (scar tissue, transection), or blood vessel disorders. The merits of duplex imaging include no intravenous contrast, lower overall cost, and no radiation exposure. However, the study can take a significant amount of time to perform. The authors' institution has had many years of success with this method and with abdomen-based microsurgical breast

reconstruction.[11] Before the advent of CTA, many authors recommended duplex ultrasound for the surgical planning of perforator flaps.

Technique

The use of color duplex ultrasound is relatively simple to establish and is often already available through an institution's vascular laboratory. Because the study can be somewhat operator-dependent, the same technician should perform the study, if possible, to ensure consistency. The patient is evaluated in the supine position, wherein a grid is drawn on the abdomen, centered over the umbilicus, and the location of the perforator is measured from the umbilicus. The donor abdomen is then divided into horizontal zones of 4-cm vertical height. A 5- to 10-MHz transducer is used with settings designed for peripheral arteries. The data are then registered on a standardized form (**Fig. 2**). The technician should evaluate the deep inferior epigastric artery; its medial and lateral branch, or the central axis if no branching occurred; perforators larger than 0.5 mm within the dimensions of the grid; and the internal mammary artery at the third intercostal space. For each of these vessels, the peak systolic flow velocity (cm/s) and vessel diameter at maximal pulsation are measured bilaterally. These data can then be translated back on the patient's abdomen at surgery, creating a map of the viable perforators (**Fig. 3**).

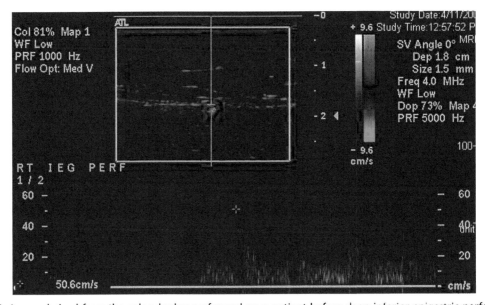

Fig. 1. Image derived from the color duplex performed on a patient before deep inferior epigastric perforator breast reconstruction showing the presence, size, and velocity of the perforator.

Philips HDI-5000 ultrasound system was utilized for this exam.

ABDOMINAL PERFORATOR ARTERIAL DUPLEX: A total of 5-right and 4-left epigastric perforators were identified and marked on the skin. Peak Systolic Velocities:

RIGHT
.... Velocity ... Diameter ... Vertical ... Horizontal
..........(cm/sec)......(cm)...........(cm).........(cm)
Zone I
     .... 56 .... 0.11 .... +2.0 .... 4.0
............51 .... 0.11 .... +1.0 .... 5.5
Zone II
     ....30 .... 0.10 .... -0.5 ....1.5
............63 .... 0.11 .... -1.0 .... 3.5
Zone III
     ...26 .... 0.10 .... -5.5 .... 2.0
Zone IV ....

LEFT

Zone I
.... 87 .... 0.13 .... +2.5 .... 1.5
.... 17 .... 0.12 .... +0.5 .... 5.0
Zone II
.... 16 .... 0.10 .... -1.5 .... 2.0
.... 13 .... 0.10 .... -3.5 .... 2.0
Zone III
....
Zone IV ....

Peak systolic velocities in the internal mammary artery are 99 cm/sec on the right and 84 cm/sec on the left. The associated veins are patent demonstrating spontaneous and phasic waveforms.

Fig. 2. A sample color duplex report. The data at the time of duplex are transposed to horizontal zones of the abdomen that are designed as 4-cm vertical areas relative to the umbilicus. The specific perforators can be plotted by coordinates from the umbilicus.

Clinical Studies with Color Duplex Ultrasound

Our institution previously relied on duplex ultrasound scanning for preoperative perforator mapping and found it to be generally accurate compared with intraoperative clinical findings.[11] It has also been studied in several series for use in perforator flaps. In their study of 32 patients undergoing deep inferior epigastric perforator (DIEP) flaps, Giunta and colleagues[12] reported that 11% of the time a perforating vessel was found intraoperatively that had been missed on preoperative Doppler. In their series of 50 consecutive DIEP flaps, Blondeel and colleagues[13] reported that color duplex scanning in planning perforator flaps yielded a high sensitivity of 96.2% and nearly a 100% positive predictive value. The map of the perforators generated by color duplex can simplify intraoperative decision making, and thereby reduce operating time. However, it cannot provide the three-dimensional information of CTA and MRA CTA.

Introduction

The introduction in 2006 by Masia and colleagues[14] of the use of the multidetector CT scanner to preoperatively map the perforators in abdomen-based microsurgical breast reconstruction showed the utility of this technique to not only locate the performator but also see the course of the underlying deep inferior epigastric artery (DIEA). During the years since this initial publication, many institutions have abandoned the use of color duplex and now routinely use CTA for the preoperative study of patients who may potentially undergo DIEP and superficial inferior epigastric artery (SIEA) breast reconstruction.[15–22] The high spatial resolution of this examination allows for multiplanar evaluation of the vessels and provides a three-dimensional view of the vessels as they travel through the rectus. These scans produce excellent anatomic images that are easy for the operating surgeon to interpret with or without the help of a radiologist. The data can

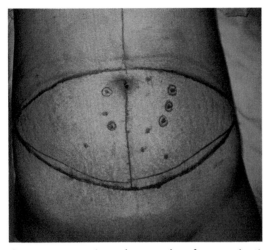

Fig. 3. Preoperative photograph of a patient's abdomen after transposition of the duplex-derived location of the perforators (*solid dots*) and those identified on CTA as the dominant perforators (*larger circles*). Although duplex located most of the perforators in this patient, it was unable to discern which ones were dominant perforators.

even be stored on a secured CD or a USB drive that can be managed with a standard computer and can be reviewed as often as necessary by the surgeon and their team.

CTA has been shown to be accurate in showing the location, size, and course of musculocutaneous perforators as small as 0.3 mm and seems to be less dependent on body habitus.[23] The scan also allows for close evaluation of the DIEA and SIEA, and their branching patterns, with high resolution. Information such as the degree to which a perforator travels within the muscle can be used in surgery to choose the dominant perforator vessels. Although these scans are useful in unilateral reconstruction, they offer significant advantage in the planning of bilateral breast reconstruction, in which the perforators chosen must supply enough tissue on each side of the abdomen to create two breast mounds, and there is less margin for error. This increased accuracy in preoperative identification of suitable vessels in patients undergoing bilateral reconstruction may thus help ensure adequate blood supply to the flaps. This information is also useful during preoperative counseling of the patient regarding the likelihood of successful bilateral DIEP flap transfer versus the need to perform muscle-sparing TRAM.

The only relative contraindications to the use of CTA are sensitivity to the intravenous contrast, severe claustrophobia (although scan times are short), and renal impairment. The major disadvantages of this technique are the radiation exposure during the examination and the cost. However, the

effective dose of radiation used in this study is 5.6 mSv, which is less than that used for a conventional abdominal CT scan.[17] A lower dose can be achieved because of the focused nature of the area scanned. However, if the surgeon requires a full chest (to evaluate the internal mammary vessels) and abdominal CTA, the radiation exposure will increase threefold.[24] The cost remains an important issue, but because preoperative imaging has been suggested to reduce operative time, this cost may be recovered during the operation.[17,25]

Technique

Patients are usually scanned using 64-slice CTA using a General Electric Lightspeed VCT Scanner (GE Healthcare, Chalfont St Giles, UK) after a target injection of 150 mL of iohexol contrast (Omnipaque 350, GE Healthcare, Chalfont St Giles, UK) at a flow rate of 4 mL/s. Axial images are processed into maximum intensity projection and reformatted into multiple views, including three-dimensional volume-rendered reconstructions using commercially available software. Located perforators are measured based on distance from the umbilicus for surgical planning.

CTA data are obtained using measurement of perforator diameter in millimeters and number of perforators in each zone; all perforators with a diameter of 1 mm or more are included in the study (**Fig. 4**). All information about the presence and size of the SIEAs is also noted (**Fig. 5**). All measured coordinates of perforator location are transposed to the abdomen with the help of three-dimensional reconstructions that seem to be highly accurate (**Fig. 6**). The reconstructions also allow for direct comparison of the surface anatomy with the underling DIEA) anatomy (**Fig. 7**). Further three-dimensional reconstructions of vessels such as the DIEAs are also routinely created (**Fig. 8**).

At the authors' institution in 2008, the approximate combined hospital and professional charges were $1734, and the study time was approximately 5 minutes, with additional time for interpretation and image reconstruction using commercially available software. The extent of scanning should be limited to the origin of the DIEA and SIEA on the common femoral as the lower limit of the scan, and the superior limit of the scan confined to the upper extent of the flap (4 cm above the umbilicus) to limit radiation exposure.

Accuracy of CTA for Locating Perforators

The accuracy of CTA was studied by Rozen and colleagues[7] in a prospective, single-blind, cohort

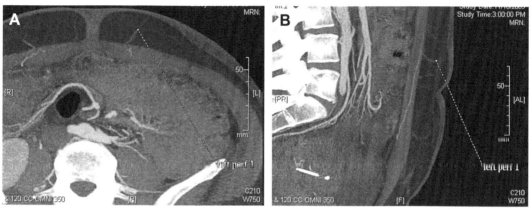

Fig. 4. CTA showing an individual perforator in both coronal (*A*) and sagittal (*B*) sections. Unlike the Doppler, this modality provides information about the course of the vessel and the location.

study of 42 patients who underwent DIEP flap surgery. They mapped all perforators larger than 1 mm both on angiography and intraoperatively using a grid of 4-mm squares centered on the umbilicus. CTA identified 280 major perforators in 42 patients; 279 perforators were identified accurately, with 1 false-positive and 1 false-negative. The sensitivity of CTA was shown to be 99.6%, with a positive predictive value of 99.6%. Therefore, the investigators concluded that CTA is highly accurate in identifying and mapping the perforators of the DIEA. Its accuracy is superior to that of the previous modalities used in this role.

CTA and Operative Time

Casey and colleagues[25] reported on their retrospective review of a consecutive series of DIEP- and SIEA-based breast reconstructions over a 5-year period. They compared operative times and postoperative outcomes in 186 flaps evaluated with hand-held Doppler versus 100 flaps evaluated with CTA imaging. The investigators found that the use of CTA resulted in a statistically significant decrease in operative times in both unilateral and bilateral cases (unilateral, 370 vs 459 minutes; bilateral, 515 vs 657 minutes; $P<.01$). CTA also identified three cases of deep inferior epigastric vessel ligation from previous operations, which compromised these as suitable source vessels. The limitations of the findings were that the study was retrospective and that the use of the Doppler was from the group's early period when they first began to use perforator flaps for breast reconstruction.

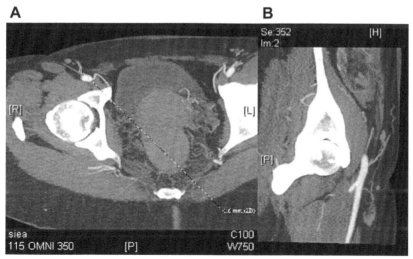

Fig. 5. Coronal (*A*) and sagittal (*B*) views can also provide valuable information about suitability of the SIEA for flaps to use in reconstruction.

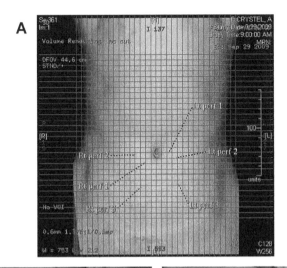

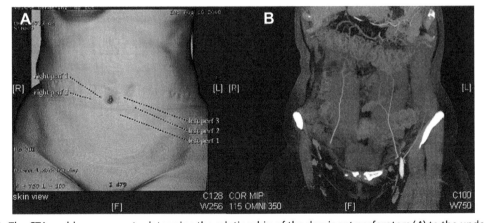

Fig. 6. (*A*) The perforators found on CTA are assembled into a three-dimensional perforator map with the overlying soft tissue, as seen in the patient's preoperative film before undergoing bilateral DIEP breast reconstruction. (*B*) These data are then transposed on the patient's abdomen, as shown in this intraoperative photo from the same patient. (*C*) The accuracy of this technique is confirmed when the perforators are dissected free, as shown in this same patient in whom a DIEP flap was harvested based on left perforator two and three located with CTA.

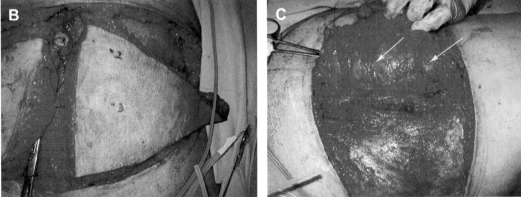

Fig. 7. The CTA enables surgeons to determine the relationship of the dominant perforators (*A*) to the underlying anatomy of the deep inferior epigastric vessels (*B*).

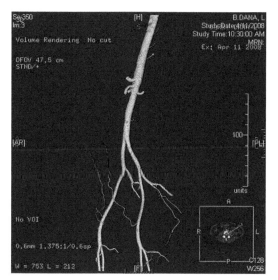

Fig. 8. A branching pattern is evident in three-dimensional reconstructions of the DIEAs.

Smit and colleagues[26] retrospectively evaluated 138 DIEP breast reconstructions, of which 70 underwent preoperative CTA analysis and 68 had preoperative Doppler investigation. Compared with the control group, the CTA group had significantly lower surgery time (264 vs 354 minutes; $P<.001$) and a tendency for fewer complications. This nonrandomized study suggested that CTA may reduce intraoperative time devoted the harvesting the flap.

Masia and colleagues[17] reported on 126 consecutive patients scheduled for postmastectomy reconstruction. In the first 36 patients, they compared the intraoperative findings with the preoperative CTA findings. In the latter 90 patients, the dominant perforator vessels were directly selected based on CTA findings. The initial study of 36 patients suggested a directed and reproducible correlation between the radiologic and intraoperative findings. In the following 90 cases, the average operating time saved per patient was 1 hour 40 minutes and there was a significant reduction in postsurgical complications. The investigators' preoperative evaluations with CTA also confirmed the wide range of variability in the vascular anatomy of the abdominal wall that has been described in other anatomic studies.

Masia and colleagues[27] recently updated their experience with preoperative imaging using CTA in 357 patients over the past 5 years. In all patients, at least one dominant perforator was identified with CTA. In 93.7% of cases, two or three potentially suitable perforators were present on each side of the abdomen; only 6.3% of cases had only one suitable perforator for flap harvest in the whole abdomen. Data analysis showed a significant decrease in the operative time necessary for flap harvest, from 3 hours and 20 minutes to 1 hour and 40 minutes, after the CTA (multidetector-row CT) was introduced into the preoperative algorithm.

CTA Versus Color Duplex Ultrasound for Preoperative Mapping of Perforators

In a recent study directly comparing CT angiography and ultrasound in eight patients, Rozen and colleagues[23] found that CTA was far superior to Doppler. However, no perforators were located in any of the eight patients who underwent duplex ultrasound, precluding any true comparison.

In a recent study directly comparing CTA with color duplex ultrasound in 23 patients, the authors found that CTA preoperatively identified 83 of the largest perforators,[28,29] and ultrasound preoperatively identified only 55 of these large perforators (66.3%). Duplex ultrasound failed to identify 28 perforators (33.7%) that CTA identified and which were later confirmed at surgery. No superficial inferior epigastric arteries were identified with ultrasound. However, in all eight breast reconstructions performed with the superficial inferior epigastric system, the surgeon or radiologist identified the SIEAs preoperatively as adequate size for microsurgical transfers, with an average diameter of 1.6 mm.

Conclusion

CTA allows surgeons the necessary anatomic data to prepare an operative strategy to harvest the best perforator. Surgeons can choose the perforator before surgery based on not only its caliber but also the route the vessels take in relationship to the muscle. This capability should enable a safer and faster flap harvest. In DIEP flap candidates who have undergone previous abdominal surgery, CTA allows excellent evaluation of postsurgical changes to the abdomen, including the viability of the DIEA system. Based on these characteristics, CTA is currently the gold standard in preoperative imaging for DIEP flaps.[30]

MRA

The most recent development in preoperative imaging for perforator-based breast reconstruction is the application of MRA. The development of MR techniques that use high field equipment and blood-pool intravascular contrast agents has allowed the performance of noninvasive and radiation-free angiographic studies of peripheral and small caliber vessels. MRA was previously validated in the preoperative evaluation of the vascular supply of the fibula.[31]

The major advantage of MR imaging over CT is the absence of ionizing radiation. The radiologist can perform multiple acquisitions during the MRA after the administration of the gadolinium-based contrast without any fear of increased exposure to radiation, as seen in CTA. This function allows the machine to obtain images of the vessels at the most optimal time. The vessel can be imaged at the moment when the signal intensity of the perforator is the highest and venous contamination is the lowest (**Fig. 9**). Although the multidetector CT seems to yield a higher spatial resolution than MR imaging, MR imaging generally yields greater contrast resolution (**Fig. 10**). The greater contrast resolution enables the detection of submillimeter gadolinium-enhanced structures, such as DIEPs (**Fig. 11A**). The technique can provide much of the same information as CTA, such as the anatomic course of the DIEP system (see **Fig. 11B**); however, some limitation in terms of intramuscular visualization of the vessels has been reported.

The disadvantages of this technique are associated with the longer duration of image acquisition and resulting length of time in the scanner, and the need for intravenous contrast. Most MRA techniques reported require the administration of Gadolinium contrast. These contrast agents can potentially induce nephrogenic systemic fibrosis (NSF), also called *nephrogenic fibrosing dermopathy*.[32,33] However, reports of NSF have been limited to patients with impaired renal function. MRA also has a higher cost than CT scanning, and several patients are unable to undergo MRA because of safety issues, such as the presence of severe claustrophobia, pacemakers, renal impairment, or implanted metal devices.

Techniques and Clinical Studies

Several studies have examined the role of MRA in preoperative imaging for perforator-based breast reconstruction. All but one have found some limitations to the technique. Alonso-Burgos and colleagues[34] sought to show the usefulness of MRA, using a 3 Tesla system for the preoperative planning for DIEP breast reconstructions. They performed MRAs on eight patients who underwent DIEP breast reconstruction, and administered 0.12 mmol/kg of gadofosveset trisodium at a rate of 1.5 mL/s, followed by a 15-mL saline flush at the same flow rate, and a scanning delay of 60 seconds after injection of contrast medium. In this small series, MRA predicted most of the main perforating vessels, with good concordance in location and vessel description conformation found at surgery. However, it missed one main perforator vessel in two of the eight patients.

Chernyak and colleagues[35] prospectively evaluated 3 Tesla gadolinium-enhanced MR imaging for localization of DIEA perforators before reconstructive breast surgery involving a DIEP flap. In this study, 19 patients underwent preoperative MR imaging of the abdominal wall. All patients received a dose (0.1 mmol per kilogram of body weight) of gadopentetate dimeglumine followed by 20 mL of normal saline solution at an injection rate of 2 mL/s. Among 30 surgical flaps, 122 perforators were localized at surgery, 118 (97%) of which—with a mean diameter of 1.1 mm (range, 0.8–1.6 mm)—had been identified at preoperative MR imaging. Among these, 30 perforators with a mean diameter of 1.4 mm (range, 1.0–1.6 mm)

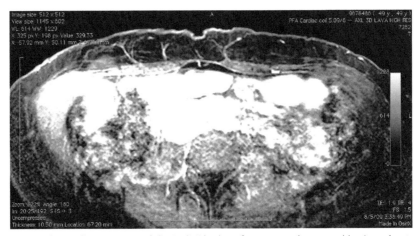

Fig. 9. MRA can provide excellent images of the individual perforators as they travel in the subcutaneous tissues. *Courtesy of* Dr David Greenspun, New York, NY.

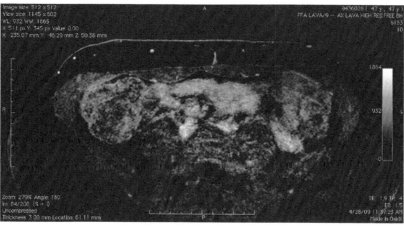

Fig. 10. MRA can even allow the surgeon to know preoperatively that one side of the abdomen is supplied by the DIEA system while the other has a SIEA-dominant blood supply. *Courtesy of* Dr David Greenspun, New York, NY.

were labeled as the best at MR imaging. A total of 33 perforators were harvested intraoperatively, all of which had been localized preoperatively, and 28 (85%) of these were labeled as the best at MR imaging.

Rozen and colleagues[36] conducted a pilot study comparing MRA with CTA and operative findings in six consecutive patients undergoing DIEP flaps for breast reconstruction. The first three patients underwent imaging using a 1.5 Tesla GE Echospeed HDx (General Electric, Milwaukee, WI, USA) scanner, and the last three patients were imaged using a 3 Tesla Siemens Magnetom Trio (Siemens Medical Solutions, Erlangen, Germany) scanner. Intravenous contrast was achieved with 30-mL Magnevist (Dimeglumine Gadopentetate; Schering, Bergkamen, Germany). The DIEA, SIEA, and perforators were all assessed with each modality in five of six patients. The investigators found that the DIEA and SIEA were accurately imaged with both CTA and MRA, but CTA was more accurate than MRA for perforator mapping. The MRA uniformly identified fewer perforators per patient than CTA. CTA also showed a greater capacity for identifying soft tissue planes, and thus the course of perforators (subcutaneous, subfacial, and intramuscular) was seen with greater accuracy.

In a recent study, Greenspun and colleagues[37] performed 3 Tesla MRA imaging with gadolinium on 31 patients who underwent 50 abdominal flaps. The investigators reported that all perforators visualized on MRA were found at surgery

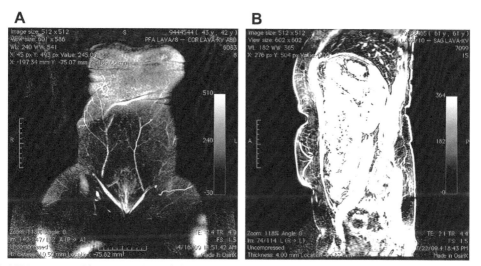

Fig. 11. MRAs can provide an overview of the DIEA system (*A*) and much of same detail as CTA on the sagittal views (*B*). *Courtesy of* Dr David Greenspun, New York, NY.

(0% false-positive). However, in 2 of 50 flaps, the surgeon transferred a flap based on a vessel not visualized on the MRA (4% false-negative). The article did not comment on issues regarding poor intramuscular visualization associated with the technique. Based on these data, the investigators believe that MRA is a reliable preoperative imaging technique for abdominal perforator flap breast reconstruction. They now use MRA as their preferred imaging modality for preoperative identification of perforators.[37]

Finally, Masia and colleagues[38] recently reported on a new technique using MRA without administering contrast. They found a 1.5 Tesla MRI acquisition sequence that provided specific vascular imaging without the use of contrast material, and tested the technique on 36 female patients undergoing breast reconstruction after mastectomy with DIEP flap. The MRA technique is based on fresh blood imaging (FBI) with a Toshiba ZGV Vantage ATLAS 1.5-T ultra–short-bore body MR system (Toshiba Medical Systems, Tokyo, Japan). This technique provided the location of the dominant perforator, definition of its intramuscular course, and the ability to evaluate the superficial inferior epigastric system.

The investigators noted that before the new technique was used, the noncontrast MRA often failed (42% of the time) to elucidate the intramuscular course of the DIEA, which has been the primary advantage of CTA over MRA. However, initial results with the MRA FBI technique show good definition of the perforator intramuscular course in all cases. This modification of the MRA technique could become a highly valuable tool in preoperative perforator mapping for DIEP flap microsurgical breast reconstruction without the need for either contrast or radiation.

MRA is still an emerging modality for imaging of DIEA perforators, which spares the patient radiation exposure and may offer an alternative to CTA in this role. Although the studies discussed earlier have shown that the perforators can be accurately imaged with MRA, CTA was still more accurate than MRA for perforator mapping and is still the preferred modality. A role for MRA in perforator imaging is suggested by these results, and based on these findings, a larger study into the role for MRA with continued refinement of MRA techniques is warranted.

SUMMARY

The recent development of radiologic techniques (CTA and MRA) that allow for improved preoperative evaluation of perforators in abdomen-based reconstruction provide surgeons with information that can reduce operative time and possibly lead to improved outcomes. The ability to evaluate the branching pattern of each perforator in the subcutaneous tissue, and then follow that perforator's course in direct relation to the muscle, enables surgeons to select the perforator that not only will perfuse the flap but also can be dissected free with the least amount of muscle dissection. Although currently CTA seems to be the gold standard for this type of evaluation, the continued refinement of MRA techniques may yield an examination that does not require the use of contrast nor any exposure to radiation.

REFERENCES

1. Blondeel PN, Boeckx WD. Refinements in free flap breast reconstruction: the free bilateral deep inferior epigastric perforator flap anastomosed to the internal mammary artery. Br J Plast Surg 1994;47(7):495.
2. Allen RJ, Treece P. Deep inferior epigastric perforator flap for breast reconstruction. Ann Plast Surg 1994;32(1):32.
3. Allen RJ. DIEP versus TRAM for breast reconstruction. Plast Reconstr Surg 2003;111(7):2478.
4. Bajaj AK, Chevray PM, Chang DW. Comparison of donor-site complications and functional outcomes in free muscle-sparing TRAM flap and free DIEP flap breast reconstruction. Plast Reconstr Surg 2006;117(3):737.
5. Blondeel N, Vanderstraeten GG, Monstrey SJ, et al. The donor site morbidity of free DIEP flaps and free TRAM flaps for breast reconstruction. Br J Plast Surg 1997;50(5):322.
6. Peeters WJ, Nanhekhan L, Van Ongeval C, et al. Fat necrosis in deep inferior epigastric perforator flaps: an ultrasound-based review of 202 cases. Plast Reconstr Surg 2009;124(6):1754.
7. Rozen WM, Ashton MW, Stella DL, et al. The accuracy of computed tomographic angiography for mapping the perforators of the DIEA: a cadaveric study. Plast Reconstr Surg 2008;122(2):363.
8. Taylor GI, Doyle M, McCarten G. The Doppler probe for planning flaps: anatomical study and clinical applications. Br J Plast Surg 1990;43(1):1.
9. Hallock GG. Doppler sonography and color duplex imaging for planning a perforator flap. Clin Plast Surg 2003;30(3):347.
10. Yu P, Youssef A. Efficacy of the handheld Doppler in preoperative identification of the cutaneous perforators in the anterolateral thigh flap. Plast Reconstr Surg 2006;118(4):928.
11. Rand RP, Cramer MM, Strandness DE Jr. Color-flow duplex scanning in the preoperative assessment of TRAM flap perforators: a report of 32 consecutive patients. Plast Reconstr Surg 1994;93(3):453.

12. Giunta RE, Geisweid A, Feller AM. The value of preoperative Doppler sonography for planning free perforator flaps. Plast Reconstr Surg 2000;105(7):2381.

13. Blondeel PN, Beyens G, Verhaeghe R, et al. Doppler flowmetry in the planning of perforator flaps. Br J Plast Surg 1998;51(3):202.

14. Masia J, Clavero JA, Larranaga JR, et al. Multidetector-row computed tomography in the planning of abdominal perforator flaps. J Plast Reconstr Aesthet Surg 2006;59(6);594.

15. Clavero JA, Masia J, Larranaga J, et al. MDCT in the preoperative planning of abdominal perforator surgery for postmastectomy breast reconstruction. AJR Am J Roentgenol 2008;191(3):670.

16. Masia J, Clavero JA, Larranaga J, et al. Preoperative planning of the abdominal perforator flap with multidetector row computed tomography: 3 years of experience. Plast Reconstr Surg 2008;122(2):80e.

17. Masia J, Larranaga J, Clavero JA, et al. The value of the multidetector row computed tomography for the preoperative planning of deep inferior epigastric artery perforator flap: our experience in 162 cases. Ann Plast Surg 2008;60(1):29.

18. Rosson GD, Williams CG, Fishman EK, et al. 3D CT angiography of abdominal wall vascular perforators to plan DIEAP flaps. Microsurgery 2007;27(8):641.

19. Rozen WM, Ashton MW, Grinsell D, et al. Establishing the case for CT angiography in the preoperative imaging of abdominal wall perforators. Microsurgery 2008;28(5):306.

20. Rozen WM, Ashton MW, Stella DL, et al. The accuracy of computed tomographic angiography for mapping the perforators of the deep inferior epigastric artery: a blinded, prospective cohort study. Plast Reconstr Surg 2008;122(4):1003.

21. Rozen WM, Phillips TJ, Ashton MW, et al. A new preoperative imaging modality for free flaps in breast reconstruction: computed tomographic angiography. Plast Reconstr Surg 2008;122(1):38e.

22. Tregaskiss AP, Goodwin AN, Bright LD, et al. Three-dimensional CT angiography: a new technique for imaging microvascular anatomy. Clin Anat 2007; 20(2):116.

23. Rozen WM, Phillips TJ, Ashton MW, et al. Preoperative imaging for DIEA perforator flaps: a comparative study of computed tomographic angiography and Doppler ultrasound. Plast Reconstr Surg 2008; 121(Supp 1):1.

24. Rozen WM, Garcia-Tutor E, Alonso-Burgos A, et al. Planning and optimising DIEP flaps with virtual surgery: the Navarra experience. J Plast Reconstr Aesthet Surg 2010;63:289–97.

25. Casey WJ III, Chew RT, Rebecca AM, et al. Advantages of preoperative computed tomography in deep inferior epigastric artery perforator flap breast reconstruction. Plast Reconstr Surg 2009;123(4):1148.

26. Smit JM, Dimopoulou A, Liss AG, et al. Preoperative CT angiography reduces surgery time in perforator flap reconstruction. J Plast Reconstr Aesthet Surg 2009;62:1112–7.

27. Masia J, Kosutic D, Clavero JA, et al. Preoperative computed tomographic angiogram for deep inferior epigastric artery perforator flap breast reconstruction. J Reconstr Microsurg 2010;26:21–8.

28. Scott JR, Liu D, Said H, et al. C.T. angiography in planning abdomen-based microsurgical breast reconstruction: a comparison to color duplex ultrasound. Plast Reconstr Surg 2010;125(2):446–53.

29. Mathes DW, Neligan PC. Current techniques in preoperative imaging for abdomen-based perforator flap microsurgical breast reconstruction. J Reconstr Microsurg 2010;26(1):3.

30. Hijjawi JB, Blondeel PN. Advancing deep inferior epigastric artery perforator flap breast reconstruction through multidetector row computed tomography: an evolution in preoperative imaging. J Reconstr Microsurg 2010;26(1):11.

31. Fukaya E, Grossman RF, Saloner D, et al. Magnetic resonance angiography for free fibula flap transfer. J Reconstr Microsurg 2007;23(4):205.

32. Dillman JR, Ellis JH, Cohan RH, et al. Frequency and severity of acute allergic-like reactions to gadolinium-containing i.v. contrast media in children and adults. AJR Am J Roentgenol 2007;189(6):1533.

33. Niendorf HP, Alhassan A, Geens VR, et al. Safety review of gadopentetate dimeglumine. Extended clinical experience after more than five million applications. Invest Radiol 1994;29(Suppl 2):S179.

34. Alonso-Burgos A, Garcia-Tutor E, Bastarrika G, et al. Preoperative planning of DIEP and SGAP flaps: preliminary experience with magnetic resonance angiography using 3-tesla equipment and blood-pool contrast medium. J Plast Reconstr Aesthet Surg 2009;63:298–304.

35. Chernyak V, Rozenblit AM, Greenspun DT, et al. Breast reconstruction with deep inferior epigastric artery perforator flap: 3.0-T gadolinium-enhanced MR imaging for preoperative localization of abdominal wall perforators. Radiology 2009;250(2):417.

36. Rozen WM, Stella DL, Phillips TJ, et al. Magnetic resonance angiography in the preoperative planning of DIEA perforator flaps. Plast Reconstr Surg 2008;122(6):222e.

37. Greenspun D, Vasile J, Levine JL, et al. Anatomic imaging of abdominal perforator flaps without ionizing radiation: seeing is believing with magnetic resonance imaging angiography. J Reconstr Microsurg 2010;26(1):37.

38. Masia J, Kosutic D, Cervelli D, et al. Search of the ideal method in perforator mapping: noncontrast magnetic resonance imaging. J Reconstr Microsurg 2010;26(1):29.

Technical Tips for Safe Perforator Vessel Dissection Applicable to All Perforator Flaps

Anne Dancey, MBChB, MmedSci, FRCS (Plast),
Phillip N. Blondeel, MD, PhD, FCCP*

KEYWORDS

- Perforator flap • Microsurgery • Flap dissection
- Operative techniques

In 1989, Koshima and Soeda[1] described a free flap that is based solely on a perforating vessel, which emanated from the deep inferior epigastric artery. Thus, it became apparent that flaps could be supplied by vessels previously dismissed as being too small to be considered. This discovery represented an evolution in flap surgery and the foundation on which a new genre of flaps was discovered.[2–8]

The principal advantage of perforator flaps is that they spare deeper structures and thus limit functional morbidity.[9–14] The size of the skin paddle that can be raised is, to a certain extent, related to the size of the perforator. Thus, inclusion of muscle has no influence on flap perfusion and it should be spared whenever possible.[15] The disadvantages of perforator flaps lie in their technical demands and the resultant potential increase in operative time. The dissection of the flap requires meticulous attention to detail and a high degree of flexibility of the operative plan according to the position, size, and presence of perforating vessels. However, the somewhat unpredictable nature of the vessels can be partly addressed by accurate preoperative imaging.

PREOPERATIVE PLANNING
Flap Planning

Accurate preoperative planning is an essential component of perforator flap surgery. Preoperative planning begins with delineation of the anatomic defect to replace "like with like". Both the dimensions and constituent parts of the defect need to be considered. Practically, this consideration can be divided into the surface area of the skin paddle, the thickness and consistency of the subcutaneous layer, the total flap volume, and any specialized structures.[16] If a complex reconstruction is necessary, the flap may need to incorporate specific anatomic components, such as bone, fascia, muscle, and nerve. The use of a perforator flap in these circumstances allows the skin flap to be mobilized from the other constituents to give flexibility in its placement. In this instance, the bone, muscle, and other such parts can be placed to permit a functional reconstruction, with the skin paddle draped to provide optimum contour. These have been termed chimeric flaps[17] and are discussed later.

Having considered what needs to be replaced, the surgeon must give consideration to the most appropriate donor site and method of flap transfer (pedicled or free). For practical purposes, it is also preferable to select a flap that does not require position changes and facilitates a 2-team approach.

Although the technical aspects of flap dissection are similar for pedicled and free flaps, there are essential differences in flap planning and raising. The epicenter of a free perforator flap must lie at the level of the feeding vessel to ensure adequate tissue perfusion to all zones.

Department of Plastic and Reconstructive Surgery, University Hospital Gent, De Pintelaan 185, Gent B-9000, Belgium
* Corresponding author. Department of Plastic and Reconstructive Surgery, University Hospital Gent, De Pintelaan 185, Gent B-9000, Belgium.
E-mail address: phillip.blondeel@ugent.be

Clin Plastic Surg 37 (2010) 593–606
doi:10.1016/j.cps.2010.06.008

Local perforator flaps offer limited flap movement around the perforator, which represents the central axis of rotation. The extent of the flap movement depends on the tissue elasticity and perforator vessel length. The latter can be increased by following the perforator into the fascia or muscle. Several studies have shown that longer pedicles are less sensitive to twisting forces, because the length of a vessel is inversely proportional to the critical angle of twisting.[18–22] Flaps that include only 1 perforator are likely to have greater flap mobility and can be mobilized in a propeller fashion, 180° counterclockwise or clockwise, without compromising perfusion. Flaps with multiple perforators are more suitable for rotational or advancement maneuvers, depending on the number of vessels preserved. If more than 1 perforator is included, then the vessels must be in close proximity to each other and dissected for a sufficient distance.

The position of the perforator selected depends on the planned movement of the flap. In a propeller flap, the perforator closest to the defect is chosen to allow the flap to pivot on the vessel and thus increase the potential coverage of the defect.[23,24] For advancement, transposition, and rotation flaps, perforators furthest from the defect are selected because this provides the longest possible pedicle thereby giving the flap a large arc of motion. Regardless of the type of flap movement, any stretching of the perforator vessels should be avoided to minimize the risk of vascular complication.

Perforator flaps can also be based on a known named perforator (in a similar manner to standard musculocutaneous or fasciocutaneous flaps) or they can be designed freestyle on a random unnamed perforator of sufficient caliber.[25]

Freestyle flaps can be considered as a form of reverse planning. The required characteristics of the skin flap determine its anatomic location, and the perforating vessels are selected as a secondary consideration. The benefits of this method lie in its flexibility in assuring that the most suitable flap is raised. However, the surgeon must be competent in locating the perforators with an ultrasound or duplex Doppler probe and must possess an excellent anatomic knowledge of the region. These flaps can be technically demanding and often require dissection and anastomosis of vessels that are considerably smaller than standard perforator flaps.

Flap design modifications and refinements

Chimeric flaps Chimeric flaps are composed of several constituent parts supplied by the same source vessel.[26] The component parts can be mobilized in relation to each other to allow a 3-dimensional reconstruction of a complex defect. The same effect can also be achieved using a flow-through flap in combination with a separate free flap, such as a flow-through anterolateral thigh flap with vascularized fibular flap.

Thin flaps It is possible to radically thin a perforator flap before transplantation. This procedure has become possible with increasing knowledge of the vascular supply of skin and subcutaneous tissue. The skin is supplied by the subdermal plexus that in turn arises from an axial vessel. Thus, it is possible to raise a thin flap without the fascia. The radical thinning should be performed in situ before the vascular pedicle is divided.[27,28] The advantage of this method of flap raising is the ability to create a flap fulfilling the exact soft tissue dimensions of the defect without the necessity for secondary flap revisions. The survival rate of these flaps is shown to be the same as conventional flaps.[29]

Innervated free flaps Although it has been shown that sensory recovery without coaptation of nerves in free flaps occurs, the recovery of pressure perception and sensation is often poor and unpredictable. Sensate reconstructions can be achieved by dissecting a sensory nerve with the perforator flap and coapting to a sensory nerve at the recipient site. This technique has been popularized in breast reconstruction and for treatment of intraoral defects. However, it is often difficult to find suitable sensory nerves at the recipient site, and the extra operative time required for nerve coaptation can be significant.[30–32]

Imaging

When designing a perforator flap, the main question of concern is how much tissue, skin, and subcutaneous fat can be harvested on one particular perforator? Regardless of whether one believes in the angiosome principle or considers vascularization to occur through a subcutaneous vascular plexus influenced by flow physiology, the toughest challenge remains the same—accurate prediction of the territory of viable tissue. This prediction is as relevant in free flaps as it is in flaps based on axial vessels. The most accurate indicator is preoperative localization of the most dominant source of blood influx by duplex Doppler or computed tomographic (CT) imaging. In addition to defining a safe flap territory, these techniques provide a degree of reassurance to the surgeon by avoiding intraoperative surprises and can considerably reduce operative time. This reduction of operative costs goes some way to offset the cost of the procedure. Magnetic resonance angiography has shown to be promising in the imaging of perforators. Not only does it produce accurate and detailed images but also, unlike CT imaging, there is no exposure to radiation.[33]

Ultrasonographic evaluation of perforator vessels

This examination is performed with a color Doppler, which uses a combination of gray-scale imaging and color Doppler imaging. This imaging modality has 100% positive predictive value with few false-negative results.[34]

Gray-scale imaging shows anatomic details for location of fixed points, axial vessels, and perforating branches. The addition of color Doppler allows identification of blood flow, direction (toward or away from probe) and pattern of flow (ie, venous or arterial), and provides a measure of blood flow velocity.[35–38]

The disadvantages of color duplex imaging are lack of showing anatomic detail and operator dependence. Color duplex imaging requires a detailed knowledge of 3-dimensional vascular anatomy and expertise in handling the device. Although this imaging provides dynamic information about blood flow, it may lead to a false sense of security. It is essential to look for vessels with a minimum size and select the largest perforator in the region of interest. This perforator selection is necessary because of the constant humeral and nervous stimuli that affect the microcirculation and thus cause fluctuations in vessel flow. Hence, flow rates do not always correlate with the size of the perforator.

In addition to preoperative imaging, it is possible to use a unidirectional handheld pencil probe for identification of superficial vessels in the operating theater. The perforators identified can be marked on the patient's skin to allow accurate flap design and aid intraoperative dissection. This is a simple and inexpensive technique, which provides a useful intraoperative adjunct.[39] However, there can be false-negative and false-positive signals as a result of interference from axial vessels or perforators that run parallel to the fascia before their suprafascial course.

CT imaging

Multidetector-row helical CT is a recent innovation that permits rapid delineation of an anatomic area of interest to give excellent resolution and low artifact rating. It takes less than 10 minutes to perform and is well tolerated by patients. This imaging technique has come into its own for identification of abdominal wall perforators.[40–42] The scanning

is performed in conjunction with an intravenous contrast medium and allows evaluation of the donor and recipient vessels. Information collected include the exact location and intramuscular course of vessels from their origin, caliber of the perforators, and identification of the dominant vessel. Delineation of the relative dominance of the deep and superficial systems removes the element of surprise and allows the surgeon to consider the options preoperatively. This modality can be used to select suitable patients preoperatively, and operative times are reduced by a mean of 21% with obvious cost benefits.[43]

The disadvantages of this modality include the x-ray dosage and use of intravenous contrast media, with a resultant risk of anaphylaxis. The x-ray dose, albeit significant, is less than a conventional liver CT scan and can be combined with staging investigations to reduce overall exposure. Interpretation is as always operator dependent, and there is an associated learning curve for the radiologist.

OPERATIVE TECHNIQUE
Perforator Flap Dissection

Perforator flaps differ from traditional free flaps in both allowing and demanding flexibility of decision making. As previously discussed, perforating vessels are dynamic structures in constant flux of flow because of varying humeral and neural stimulations. The direct visualization of these perforators allows an assessment of caliber not afforded by static preoperative imaging. The vessel diameters and the proportionate size of the vessel must be assessed in relation to the flap dimensions. A small flap from the extremities would be well perfused by a perforator of 1 mm caliber, whereas in the deep inferior epigastric artery perforator (DIEAP) or superior gluteal artery perforator (SGAP) flap, this caliber would be considered insufficient. The surgeon must consider not only the main perforating vessel but also the adjacent perforators. Pre- and intraoperative delineation of these additional vessels allow the viable boundaries of the flap to be established and thus potentially avoid flap necrosis.

Incision and approach of the perforator
The surgeon begins by incising the edge of the skin flap. Initially, only one skin edge is incised to permit alteration of the skin paddle according to the feeding vessel selected. When mobilizing the flap and approaching the main pedicle, several additional subcutaneous vessels of more than 0.5 mm in diameter should be preserved (**Fig. 1**). These additional vessels can be dissected to

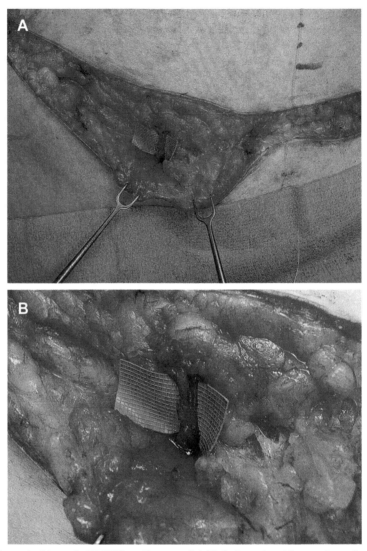

Fig. 1. (*A*) At the lower incision of a DIEAP flap, the superficial inferior epigastric vessels can be located, if present and of sufficient caliber, somewhere halfway in the inguinal ligament. (*B*) Detailed image shows the artery lateral to the superficial epigastric vein.

a reasonable length for anastomosis (often in the order of 1–4 cm) in case they are required at a later stage to augment arterial or venous flow. The flap can be beveled as necessary to provide additional tissue, with minimization of the skin paddle and donor site defect.

The dissection proceeds at either the suprafascial or subfascial level, depending on the flap being raised and surgeon preference. Small vessels can be identified within the flap as the dissection proceeds and these can be followed until they converge on the vessel of origin. The surgeon can use loupe magnification to assist in identification of vessels. Several intraoperative factors indicate the caliber of the perforator

encountered. Factors include the size of the converging branches, whether the perforators have any visible pulsation, and also the extent of the facial opening traversed by the perforator. Larger fascial openings tend to be associated with larger perforators, even if this is not immediately apparent because of vessel spasm. It is crucial to approach the vessels in a blood-free environment because this assists in identifying the converging prefascial branches. Furthermore, the relative transparency of the subcutaneous fat allows the approximate location of the perforator to be viewed in advance (**Fig. 2**), thus avoiding inadvertent damage. Blood-free clean dissection can be achieved by separating the tissue with

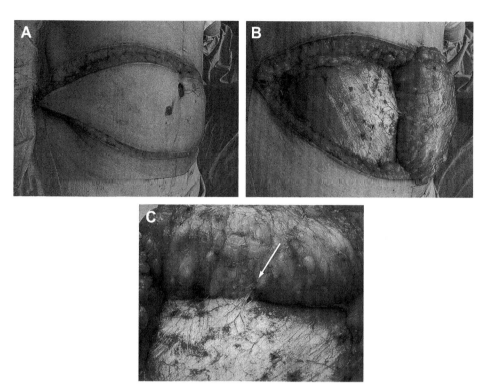

Fig. 2. (*A*) The "x" on the flap indicates the position of the most dominant perforator on the right side of the DIEAP flap. (*B*) This "x" corresponds to the area where the perforator pierces through the deep fascia. (*C*) A slit in the deep fascia and a blue hue shining through the subcutaneous fat indicates the exact location of the perforator (*arrow*).

low-current electrocautery and a wide spatula tip. It is essential to preserve all perforating vessels until a more dominant vessel is encountered. This precaution avoids the inadvertent transection of a dominant perforator that would compromise perfusion. If more than one perforator is to be included in the flap, then the perforators can be approached from different directions to allow simultaneous dissection and identification. The inclusion of multiple perforators must not sacrifice muscle or divide important motor nerves, which would negate the advantages of raising a perforator flap. If it is essential to divide a motor nerve then it must be surgically repaired. It is at this stage in flap dissection that accurate preoperative imaging allows speedier vessel dissection and sacrifice of nondominant vessels before reaching the predetermined dominant perforator.

Dealing with the deep fascia

Once the perforator has been identified and approached in the prefascial plane, further undermining should be performed between the subcutaneous fat and deep fascia for a distance of 2 to 4 cm around the perforator (**Fig. 3**). It is crucial to

perform this step before opening the deep fascia because once the fascia has been breached, the dissection becomes increasingly difficult to execute. In addition, the step provides an easily visible safety zone around the perforator, thus helping to avoid potential damage to the vessel when the remaining flap is lifted off the deep fascia in the final phase of dissection.

Once a clear circumferential view of the perforator has been established, it is necessary to open the deep fascia and follow the vessel through its intramuscular course. Opening the fascia is considerably easier if the fascial opening is large. The collagenous cuff around the perforator is cut and opened with specially designed fine scissors (Blondeel scissors, S&T AG, Neuhausen, Switzerland) until the loose connective tissue around the perforator is encountered (**Fig. 4**). While moving and contracting, the loose connective tissue allows the perforator to glide between the muscle fibers and tendinous inscriptions of the rectus abdominis muscle. Dissection close to the vessels and within this loose connective tissue facilitates liberation of the vessels in a bloodless environment. Small fascial openings are often

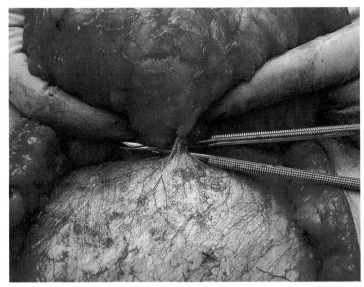

Fig. 3. Lifting the fat off the deep fascia about 2 cm around the perforator at this phase makes dissection easier.

closely adherent to the perforator. In this situation, it may be necessary to incise the deep fascia lateral to the perforator and identify the immediate intramuscular course and then leave a cuff of fascia around the vessel. When incising the fascia, it is important to realize that the perforator may run obliquely under the fascia before diving into the muscle. Hence, diligence is required to avoid inadvertent damage to the vessel.

In certain flaps, the perforators can be approached from underneath the deep fascia, such as in the SGAP flap. In such situations, a safe and slow approach to the perforator is hampered by the presence of thick epimysia that need to be cut throughout their entire length. By selecting a subfascial approach, the

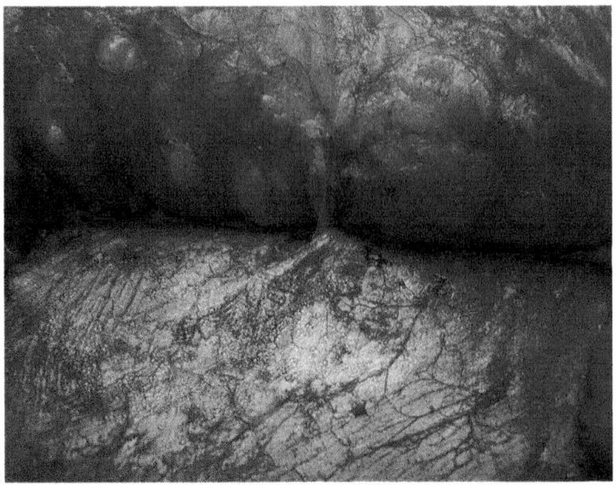

Fig. 4. Incising the collagenous cuff around the vessels exposes the gap in the deep fascia and frees the perforator.

perforator can be easily identified because of the transparent epimysia.

After identifying the main perforator below the deep fascia and just before entering the muscle or septum, the same circumferential dissection around the perforator should be done as above the fascia (**Fig. 5**). This space is avascular and filled with loose collagenous tissue, so dissection advances easily. In this case, it is also important to release the remaining attachments of the deep fascia to the perivascular tissue cuff, freeing the perforator entirely above the muscle.

The intramuscular dissection

Once the initial incision of the fascia is made cranial and caudal to the perforator, the fascia can be opened to achieve better exposure. This step can be done in any direction but is preferentially performed in the same direction as the underlying muscle fibers and toward, or over, the main supplying deep vessels (see **Fig. 5**). It is crucial to incise the deep fascia as much as necessary to gain wide exposure of the vessels in the surgical field. The opening of the fascia leaves no donor site morbidity (provided proper resuturing is performed), whereas an inadequate exposure risks damaging of the vessel. At the point where the perforator enters the muscle, the muscle fibers are split in both directions by blunt dissection (**Fig. 6**). The loose connective tissue cuff around the vessels guides the path through the muscle and indicates where the muscle fibers need to be split. In a first phase, the muscle fibers on top of the perforator and the axial vessels are split to expose the course of the pedicle through the

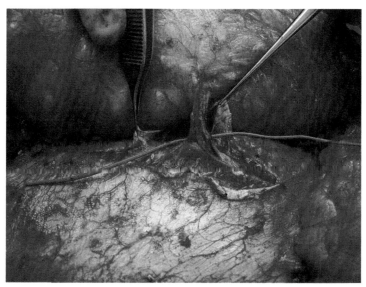

Fig. 5. Incising the deep fascia above and below the perforator and circumferential dissection around the perforator below the deep fascia give a good view on the size and caliber of the vessels.

muscle. This so-called deroofing process allows quick visual inspection of the pedicle to confirm its patency and valid vessel size, allows for early and quick adjustments to the intraoperative surgical strategy, but most of all allows wide exposure and thus good visualization of the entire pedicle (**Fig. 7**).

Intramuscular dissection requires a meticulous technique to identify the main vessels and ligate any side branches. Accidental rupture, damage,

or division of these branches results in bleeding, which obscures the operative view and risks damage to the vessels while achieving hemostasis. It is therefore essential to maintain a bloodless field at all times. Hemostasis should be secured with bipolar cautery or by clipping larger vessels, while constantly irrigating with warm saline to ensure that there is an adequate view of the vessel. Every side branch should be coagulated, ligated, or clipped at least 1 to 2 mm away

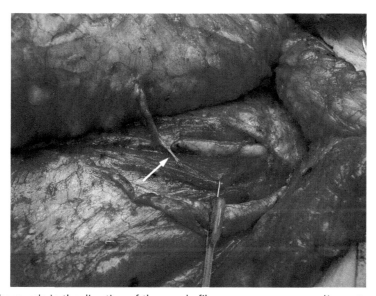

Fig. 6. Splitting the muscle in the direction of the muscle fibers exposes sensory and/or motor nerves (*arrow*).

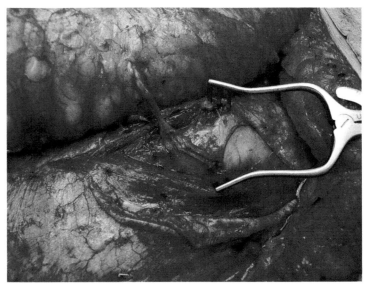

Fig. 7. Deroofing the vessels indicates the proper course and direction to the axial vessels.

from the perforator to avoid damage to the vessel and allow hemostasis to be resecured if there is continued bleeding.

Adequate exposure is also essential and is achieved with the use of self-retaining retractors or elastic retractor hooks (5 mm Sharp Hook Elastic Stays; Lone Star Medical Products, Houston, TX, USA). These retractors consist of a metal hook attached to a length of elastic. The hook retracts the tissue while tension is maintained by securing the elastic to a drape or skin staple. Retractors allow surgical instrumentation within the operative field to be kept to a minimum and free the surgical assistant for performing diathermy and irrigation. The perforator is always kept under direct vision to ensure that there is no tension on the vessel during flap manipulations and that it does not become desiccated. Securing the flap to the patient with staples or sutures should help prevent such inadvertent damage.

Direct handling of the vessels should be avoided, and while the perforators are completely freed from the surrounding tissue, the direction of dissection should always be sweeping away from the vessel itself. The dissection plane is at the level of the loose connective tissue layer that surrounds the vessels. This layer can be easily freed by blunt dissection, and any resistance encountered indicates a side branch. The instruments used for dissection are a matter of surgeon preference, but it is the authors' practice to use bipolar diathermy forceps and dissection scissors,

such as the Blondeel dissection scissors. The ring handle configuration of these scissors makes them suitable for preparation of fine structures, while the additional round handle and spring instrument configuration of the curved blades is extremely useful for fine trimming and dissection work. Once the larger deeper vessel is reached, dissection proceeds until sufficient caliber and length are achieved (**Fig. 8**).

The main pedicle

Nerves will often be encountered at the level of the deeper vessels, often just underneath or within the deeper part of the muscle (see **Fig. 6**). Depending on the region of dissection, nerves can be classified as sensory, motor, or both. Adequate anatomic knowledge and nerve stimulators can help differentiate between these different fibers. Sensory nerves to the flap can be used to reanastomose to recipient sensory nerves. The length of the donor nerve can be increased as necessary by retrograde dissection. Motor nerves are dissected off the vessels over an adequate length to allow easy dissection of the vessels underneath. These nerves are always accompanied with one or more vascular side branches that need to be clipped. Occasionally, it is necessary to divide the motor nerve. In such circumstances, a quick reanastomosis can be performed with two 9-0 nylon stitches in the perineurium. This procedure is performed once the flap has been harvested or moved.

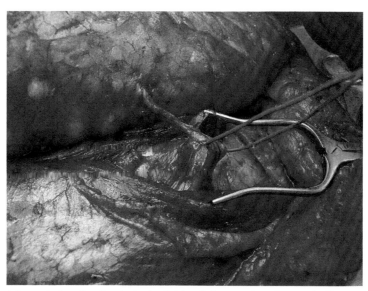

Fig. 8. Once the axial vessels are visualized, the backside of the vessels is dissected off the surrounding tissues.

In a free perforator flap, dissection of the main vessel continues until an adequate pedicle length has been achieved to perform easy anastomosis. It is equally important to reach a donor vessel diameter that is suitable in size for the recipient vessels. Good interaction between the 2 teams harvesting the flap and preparing the recipient site saves valuable operative time and permits simultaneous identification and characterization of the recipient vessels. Often 1 artery and 2 comitant veins are included in the pedicle. The smallest comitant vein is immediately ligated at the end of the dissection of the pedicle to redirect and precondition flow into the larger vein. Transection of the vein is preferentially done immediately downstream of a branch interconnecting both comitant veins, the so-called H-connectors. Although multiple H-connectors exist over the entire pedicle, anastomosis at this site allows easy flow over the anastomosis. A good anastomosis of 1 vein is preferred over linking 2 veins to ensure appropriate venous flow.

Pedicled perforator flaps are planned as rotation, advancement, or transpositional flaps. The flaps may include one or more perforating vessels. However, flaps that include only one perforator offer increased freedom of movement without vascular compromise.[25]

Once the feeding vessel has been identified, dissection of the vessel is continued as long as necessary to allow tension-free positioning of the flap in the recipient site's defect. Tracing the perforator to its original source vessel is not always necessary once sufficient flap mobility is obtained.

The aim is that when the flap is in the recipient site, there will be a degree of redundancy in the vessels, which ensures that there is no tension on the perforator, even when subjected to postoperative swelling or hematoma.

Rotation flap In this situation, the dominant perforator acts as a pivot point. The flap is designed in the fashion of a propeller blade. The longest part of the flap turns approximately180° into the defect. Dissection of the perforator is often over a short distance but long enough to ensure that turning of the flap does not cause torsion of the vessel to the extent that it compromises perfusion. To sufficiently liberate the pedicle, the distance between the end of the dissection and the entry point in the flap needs to be slightly shortened. In that way, the vein is allowed to gently turn around the artery.

Advancement flap In this case, the flap is simply slid in one direction, parallel to the direction of the muscle fibers. Dissection can go down to the axial vessels, which occasionally also require mobilization. An oblique course of the vessels to the skin surface is needed to allow movement of the flap. The longer the perforator the more the movement of the flap. Any design of skin island can be used, provided the limits of viability are respected.

Transposition flap For further displacements, a longer leash is necessary. Movements of displacement, advancement, and rotation are performed simultaneously. Sufficient slack of the pedicle is necessary without causing kinking of the pedicle. It is essential to plan accurately and take exact measurements before making skin incisions. The size of the skin island is, once again, determined by the limit of blood flow to the periphery of the flap. Therefore, a central location of the perforator in the flap is preferred. It is also important to avoid subcutaneous tunneling of flaps in areas of dense subcutaneous tissues, such as the sacral and gluteal area. Subcutaneous tunneling may compromise perfusion, resulting in fat necrosis or in the worst instance, flap loss.

Recipient Vessel Selection and Preparation

Characteristics of the ideal recipient vessels include nontraumatized, nonscarred, nonirradiated, and disease free (at least 1 artery and 1 vein) with a sufficient length to perform easy microanastomosis and a diameter that corresponds to the donor vessels. Traumatized or irradiated vessels are difficult to expose, resulting in considerable risk of iatrogenic trauma and higher rates of thrombosis and flap failure. For some conventional free flaps, an interposition graft may be required to lengthen the flap pedicle and allow anastomosis out with the zone of injury. Many studies have shown the use of such grafts increases the rate of flap failure.[44–47]

Unlike conventional free flaps, perforator flaps have consistently longer vascular pedicles that give them the increased flexibility for anastomosis to most recipient vessels. Thus, using a perforator flap can ensure that the most appropriate recipient vessels are selected to maximize the chance of flap success. The only limitation is the size of the flap vessels, which may necessitate an end-to-side anastomosis—the use of perforator recipient vessels or anastomosis to the side branch of a large recipient vessel. In supermicrosurgery, a perforator-to-perforator anastomosis that eliminates the need to dissect the flap vessels down to the larger axial vessels is performed. Such an anastomosis not only increases the ease of dissection but also makes the size of vessels more compatible. Although this may seem like an obvious progression, it should be remembered that usage of even smaller vessel diameters increases the risk of thrombosis and flap failure.[48–50]

Preparation of the recipient vessels requires the same meticulous technique as flap raising. Hemostasis must be controlled by vascular clips or bipolar coagulation and aided by irrigation. Perivascular hematoma has been shown to cause vasospasm and flow disturbances, as well as prolonging vessel wall ischemia with resultant increased inflammatory response.[51]

Exposure of the vessel should be wide to facilitate dissection and prevent compression of the pedicle against adjacent structures. Most part of the vessel dissection is performed under loupe magnification, with the final stages sometimes requiring an operating microscope, especially in a case of perforator-to-perforator anastomosis. The key to vessel dissection is advancement in the perivascular plane between the vessel and its vascular sheath. Once the sheath is divided, it can be retracted by gentle pulling and is then removed. The vessel is then sharply divided and the adventitia is trimmed. It is important to facilitate the anastomosis as much as possible by preparing the field adequately. A green or blue background is placed behind the vessel to be anastomosed, keeping all other structures out of the way. Continuous low–negative-pressure microsuction can be secured under the background using a small drain held with staples. Skin retraction is achieved with the autoretractors mentioned earlier. The flap is secured atraumatically in a suitable position by wrapping it in a saline-soaked gauze and stapling the gauze to the skin around the recipient site. All these maneuvers free the assistant to help with vessel preparation. Irrigation is performed with normal saline or heparin solution (50,000 U in 500 mL lactated Ringer solution)[52,53] as long as the intima is exposed. Either the artery or the vein can be repaired first, and the sequence is often determined by vessel position rather than an optimal order. Vessels located in deeper planes or furthest away from the surgeon's hands are sutured first. Two venous anastomoses may seem to be an obvious option if there is any doubt about venous outflow. However, caution should be exercised as this potentially reduces the venous outflow in each vessel and can lead to sludging and thrombosis.[54]

COMPLICATIONS AND LIMITATIONS

As with all promising techniques, there is a steep learning curve,[55] and the perforator flap is by no means an exception. This learning curve is composed of 3 main elements.[56]

The first is the surgical technique itself, which is experience dependent. In inexperienced hands, the dissection of small vessels through muscle can be difficult, tedious, and time consuming. However, once a surgeon has reached the plateau of the learning curve, it has been shown that the mean time for a DIEAP flap can be significantly less than a transverse rectus abdominis myocutaneous flap.[57] Good preoperative planning with the aid of angio-CTs, operating in a bloodless field, and creating wide exposure are the key elements for a complication-free and swift operation. Double operating teams obviously cut down on operative time significantly.

The second element is the experience and organization of the operating staff. It is essential to have a strong support team both in theater and on the wards, who have good clinical experience and ensure the smooth running of the surgery and follow-up. The best way to maximize flap salvage is to ensure early detection of postoperative problems in blood circulation by the staff and to undertake prompt and decisive action to reexplore the vessels as soon as possible. A flap is mainly lost when a surgeon decides to wait and observe for too long. In case of doubt, the flap is taken back to the operating room and explored.

The third component is also referred to as the pendulum effect. The introduction of a new technique results in much excitement and enthusiasm. The surgeon is inclined to apply the technique excessively, even in cases that would be better served with an alternative procedure. Having gained personal insight into the difficulties of the procedure, the pendulum swings back to the neutral position, and the surgeon uses the flap when the indications are optimum.

Preoperative imaging aids greatly in the prediction of problems and can allow modification of the surgical plan to avoid these pitfalls. Even with this reassurance, surgeons should avoid completely circumscribing the flap until they have localized the main perforator and ensured that the flap is centered on this vessel. With a limited-incision technique, the flap design can thus be modified, converted to a conventional myocutaneous technique, or even abandoned and directly closed without unnecessary sacrifice of tissue.

The key to success in perforator surgery is to avoid irreparable damage anticipating potential problems and saving any anastomosable vessel for such an event. For example, if venous or arterial compromise becomes evident with a single perforator or a superficial vascular system, then additionally prepared vessels can be anastomosed to other recipient vessels to augment blood flow. The size of the perforator selected is of extreme significance and is closely correlated to the size of the flap it perfuses. For large flaps such as a DIEAP or SGAP, the size of the concomitant perforating vein should be at least 1 mm. The artery can be much smaller than the vein, but it needs to deliver sufficient antegrade blood flow and retrograde venous return. It is difficult to advise about the absolute size and diameter of the vessels. Large and thick flaps need and mostly have large perforators. Small thin flaps can survive perfectly well on a very small pedicle. Perforators

in the same anatomic area can vary in size from one patient to the other, depending on their body habitus. Multiple studies have shown that patients with a higher body mass index have larger perforators. An ideal patient is the one who has lost a significant amount of weight because the size of the perforators is maintained after weight reduction. So, instead of looking for absolute figures for diameters, it is advised to look for relative sizes comparing different perforators in the same area. The largest of these perforators is most often the dominant. The dominant perforator can always be harvested with an additional perforator localized close to, or within, the same epimysium as the main perforator.

It is important to make the dissection as simple as possible. Perforators can course through the septum or have a short or protracted intramuscular course. If there are similar-sized perforators then those requiring the simplest dissection should be selected. In addition, the surgeon should consider the proximity of motor nerves. Crossover or adherence of these nerves to the perforator may also serve to make the dissection more tedious.

When the flap has been dissected, the surgeon should avoid transecting the secondary perforators until the dominant vessel has been dissected to its origin and the flap is ready for anastomosis. The flap should be constantly secured to the patient, and attention should be paid to the perforator to ensure that it is not placed under any tension. Although strict adherence to these guidelines should prevent accidental damage, should this occur, the flap can be raised on a contralateral perforator or as a myocutaneous flap.

The success rate of perforator flaps is directly related to the experience of the microsurgeon. The small size of the pedicle combined with the absence of a muscular cuff to protect the vessels makes the anastomosis more vulnerable to injury. Dissection of vessels often results in vasospasm. However, the mechanical effect of adventitial stripping often causes compensatory vasodilation by interrupting the sympathetic supply and mechanically thinning the walls. Unless the vessels are abnormal (eg, perivascular fibrosis), it is highly unlikely that vascular spasm will persist to the extent it causes permanent flap damage. If this spasm persists after 30 minutes or more, the addition of papaverine (an opium alkaloid acting through smooth muscle) can help to alleviate the problem. Still, if there is failure to achieve a satisfactory arterial input to the flap when the patient is physiologically optimized (flow is predominantly influenced by the mean arterial blood pressure), then the failure is most likely to be the result of an inadequate anastomosis, flap dissection error, or arterial problems proximal to the anastomosis. The surgeon should ensure that there is flow in the proximal feeding artery and that there is no kinking, twisting, or tension. The site of clamp application should be examined for damage to the vessel wall. If the proximal flow is adequate, then the anastomosis should be inspected and resected completely. The flap should be thoroughly washed through with urokinase, streptokinase, or plasminogen activator.[58–60] Direct injection of these agents into the artery, with the venous outflow left open to drain in the operating field, prevents the systemic side effects of an intravenous infusion and allows toxins to be washed out of the vein. If the vessel is heavily thrombosed, it should not be used and another flap or recipient site vessel should be explored. The use of interposition grafts may be necessary.

The venous system is more fragile than the arterial system because of the thinner walls and low flow conditions. This fragility makes them more sensitive to kinking or torsion, unlike the arterial system. Venous insufficiency of a perforator flap can be caused by inadequate drainage of the concomitant vein, and this insufficiency is sometimes seen when the superficial system is dominant and the perforators are of a small caliber. In such an event, there are several options available to the surgeon[56]:

1. *Use of the superficial veins preserved during dissection.* If an adequate length of vein has already been preserved, it can be anastomosed directly to the recipient vessels or to an additional recipient vessel to augment the flow. If the length of the vessel is inadequate then an interposition graft can be used. Arterial interposition grafts are preferred to vein grafts because they are stiffer and maintain patency of the vein, resulting in less vascular impedance to flow.
2. A second arterial or venous perforator can be anastomosed to a side branch of the main vascular pedicle.
3. *A superficial vein on the ipsilateral side can be attached to the main vascular pedicle.* This procedure can be done in an end-to-side or end-to-end fashion with a side branch and may require the use of an interposition graft.
4. The addition of an anastomosis across the midline of the flap between the 2 deep systems.
5. Anastomosis of a superficial vein to an additional vein at the recipient site.

No-flow phenomenon occurs when tissue fails to perfuse adequately, despite a patent arterial anastomosis. There is a progressive obstruction to blood flow with increasing ischemic time, which is thought to be due to cellular swelling, leakage of intravascular fluid, and intravascular aggregation and stagnation with sludging and thrombus formation. One other factor that could influence the no-flow phenomenon is microemboli that form after a microvascular anastomosis. The fate of these emboli remains unclear, but they may well be responsible for flap ischemia.[61]

SUMMARY

In the last 30 years, free flap surgery has become routine for most plastic surgeons. However, the introduction of perforator flaps met with much animosity in the surgical community, challenging conventional teaching and often branded as being unsafe. Surgeries using perforator flaps are now routinely and safely practiced all over the world, with increasing emphasis on minimizing donor site morbidity to become the current gold standard in reconstruction.

The simple principles and techniques of perforator dissection can be applied to all perforator flaps, provided the surgeon has an intimate knowledge of the regional anatomy. This knowledge has enabled a whole new field of freestyle perforator flaps to emerge.[62,63] More than 400 perforator vessels are present in the human body, and even the smallest of these vessels can now be dissected to harvest virtually any piece of skin that incorporates a feeding vessel. Further developments in this field are awaited that will shape the future of plastic surgery.

REFERENCES

1. Koshima I, Soeda S. Inferior epigastric artery skin flap without rectus abdominis muscle. Br J Plast Surg 1989;42(6):645–8.
2. Koshima I, Soeda S, Yamasaki M, et al. The free or pedicled anteromedial thigh flap. Ann Plast Surg 1988;21(5):480–5.
3. Koshima I, Moriguchi T, Soeda S, et al. Free thin paraumbilical perforator-based flaps. Ann Plast Surg 1992;29(1):12–7.
4. Koshima I, Soeda S. Free posterior tibial perforator-based flaps. Ann Plast Surg 1991;26(3):284–8.
5. Kroll SS, Rosenfield L. Perforator-based flaps for low posterior midline defects. Plast Reconstr Surg 1988; 81(4):561–6.
6. Zhou G, Qiao Q, Chen GY, et al. Clinical experience and surgical anatomy of 32 free anterolateral thigh flap transplantations. Br J Plast Surg 1991;44(2): 91–6.
7. Itoh Y, Arai K. The deep inferior epigastric artery free skin flap: anatomic study and clinical application.

Plast Reconstr Surg 1993;91(5):853–63 [discussion: 864].

8. Blondeel PN, Boeckx WD. Refinements in free flap breast reconstruction: the free bilateral deep inferior epigastric perforator flap anastomosed to the internal mammary artery. Br J Plast Surg 1994; 47(7):495–501.

9. Blondeel N, Vanderstraeten GG, Monstrey SJ, et al. The donor site morbidity of free DIEAP flaps and free TRAM flaps for breast reconstruction. Br J Plast Surg 1997;50(5):322–30.

10. Blondeel N, Boeckx WD, Vanderstraeten GG, et al. The fate of the oblique abdominal muscles after free TRAM flap surgery. Br J Plast Surg 1997; 50(5):315–21.

11. Nahabedian MY, Dooley W, Singh N, et al. Contour abnormalities of the abdomen after breast reconstruction with abdominal flaps: the role of muscle preservation. Plast Reconstr Surg 2002;109(1):91–101.

12. Nahabedian MY, Manson PN. Contour abnormalities of the abdomen after transverse rectus abdominis muscle flap breast reconstruction: a multifactorial analysis. Plast Reconstr Surg 2002;109(1):81–7 [discussion: 88–90].

13. Futter CM, Webster MH, Hagen S, et al. A retrospective comparison of abdominal muscle strength following breast reconstruction with a free TRAM or DIEAP flap. Br J Plast Surg 2000;53(7): 578–83.

14. Hamdi M, Decorte T, Demuynck M, et al. Shoulder function after harvesting a thoracodorsal artery perforator flap. Plast Reconstr Surg 2008;122(4): 1111–7 [discussion: 1118–9].

15. Angrigiani C, Grilli D, Siebert J. Latissimus dorsi musculocutaneous flap without muscle. Plast Reconstr Surg 1995;96(7):1608–14.

16. Blondeel P, Ali R. Planning of perforator flaps. In: Blondeel PN, Morris SF, Hallock GG, et al, editors. Perforator flaps: anatomy, technique & clinical applications. St Louis (MO): Quality Medical Pub; 2005. p. 109–12.

17. Hallock GG. Further clarification of the nomenclature for compound flaps. Plast Reconstr Surg 2006; 117(7):151e–60e.

18. Bilgin SS, Topalan M, Chow SP. Effect of torsion on microvenous anastomotic patency in a rat model and early thrombolytic phenomenon. Microsurgery 2003;23:381–6.

19. Selvaggi G, Anicic S, Formaggia L. Mathematical explanation of the buckling of the vessels after twisting of the microanastomosis. Microsurgery 2006;26:524–8.

20. Salgarello M, Lahoud P, Selvaggi G, et al. The effect of twisting on microanastomotic patency of arteries and veins in a rat model. Ann Plast Surg 2001;47: 643–6.

21. Topalan M, Bilgin SS, Chow SP. Effect of torsion on microarterial anastomosis patency. Microsurgery 2003;23:56–9.

22. Demir A, Acar M, Yldz L, et al. The effect of twisting on perforator flap viability: an experimental study in rats. Ann Plast Surg 2006;56:186–9.

23. Hyakusoku H, Yamamoto T, Fumiiri M. The propeller flap method. Br J Plast Surg 1991;44(1):53–4.

24. Hallock GG. The propeller flap version of the adductor muscle perforator flap for coverage of ischial or trochanteric pressure sores. Ann Plast Surg 2006;56(5):540–2.

25. Bravo FG, Schwarze HP. Free-style local perforator flaps: concept and classification system. J Plast Reconstr Aesthet Surg 2009;62(5):602–8.

26. Hallock GG. Simultaneous transposition of anterior thigh muscle and fascia flaps: an introduction to the chimera flap principle. Ann Plast Surg 1991; 27(2):126–31.

27. Kimura N, Saitoh M, Okamura T, et al. Concept and anatomical basis of microdissected tailoring method for free flap transfer. Plast Reconstr Surg 2009; 123(1):152–62.

28. Kimura N, Satoh K, Hosaka Y. Microdissected thin perforator flaps: 46 cases. Plast Reconstr Surg 2003;112(7):1875–85.

29. Ohjimi H, Taniguchi Y, Kawano K, et al. A comparison of thinning and conventional free-flap transfers to the lower extremity. Plast Reconstr Surg 2000; 105(2):558–66.

30. Blondeel PN. The sensate free superior gluteal artery perforator (S-GAP) flap: a valuable alternative in autologous breast reconstruction. Br J Plast Surg 1999;52(3):185–93.

31. Kimata Y, Uchiyama K, Ebihara S, et al. Comparison of innervated and noninnervated free flaps in oral reconstruction. Plast Reconstr Surg 1999;104(5): 1307–13.

32. Yap LH, Whiten SC, Forster A, et al. The anatomical and neurophysiological basis of the sensate free TRAM and DIEAP flaps. Br J Plast Surg 2002; 55(1):35–45.

33. Alonso-Burgos A, García-Tutor E, Bastarrika G, et al. Preoperative planning of DIEP and SGAP flaps: preliminary experience with magnetic resonance angiography using 3-tesla equipment and blood-pool contrast medium. J Plast Reconstr Aesthet Surg 2010;63(2):298–304.

34. Dirk VAM, Petrovic M. Ultrasound evaluation of perforator vessels. In: Blondeel PN, Morris SF, Hallock GG, et al, editors. Perforator flaps: anatomy, technique & clinical applications. St Louis (MO): Quality Medical Pub; 2005. p. 92–102.

35. Giunta RE, Geisweid A, Feller AM. The value of preoperative Doppler sonography for planning free perforator flaps. Plast Reconstr Surg 2000;105(7): 2381–6.

36. Hallock GG. Doppler sonography and color duplex imaging for planning a perforator flap [review]. Clin Plast Surg 2003;30(3):347–57, v–vi.

37. Iida H, Ohashi I, Kishimoto S, et al. Preoperative assessment of anterolateral thigh flap cutaneous perforators by colour Doppler flowmetry. Br J Plast Surg 2003;56(1):21–5.

38. Pacifici A, Tinti A, Flamini FO, et al. Colour flow duplex scanning: an accurate, non-invasive technique for preoperative evaluation of the vascular supply of the rectus abdominis myocutaneous flap. Scand J Plast Reconstr Surg Hand Surg 1995; 29(4):319–24.

39. Blondeel PN, Beyens G, Verhaeghe R, et al. Doppler flowmetry in the planning of perforator flaps. Br J Plast Surg 1998;51(3):202–9.

40. Masia J, Clavero JA, Larrañaga JR, et al. Multidetector-row computed tomography in the planning of abdominal perforator flaps. J Plast Reconstr Aesthet Surg 2006;59(6):594–9.

41. Masia J, Larrañaga J, Clavero JA, et al. The value of the multidetector row computed tomography for the preoperative planning of deep inferior epigastric artery perforator flap: our experience in 162 cases. Ann Plast Surg 2008;60(1):29–36.

42. Rozen WM, Garcia-Tutor E, Alonso-Burgos A, et al. Planning and optimising DIEAP flaps with virtual surgery: the Navarra experience. J Plast Reconstr Aesthet Surg 2010;63(2):289–97.

43. Uppal RS, Casaer B, Van Landuyt K, et al. The efficacy of preoperative mapping of perforators in reducing operative times and complications in perforator flap breast reconstruction. J Plast Reconstr Aesthet Surg 2009;62(7):859–64.

44. Miller MJ, Schusterman MA, Reece GP, et al. Interposition vein grafting in head and neck reconstructive microsurgery. J Reconstr Microsurg 1993;9(3): 245 51 [discussion: 251–2]

45. Yazar S. Selection of recipient vessels in microsurgical free tissue reconstruction of head and neck defects [review]. Microsurgery 2007;27(7):588–94.

46. Suominen S, Asko-Seljavaara S. Free flap failures. Microsurgery 1995;16(6):396–9.

47. Bayramiçli M, Tetik C, Sönmez A, et al. Reliability of primary vein grafts in lower extremity free tissue transfers. Ann Plast Surg 2002;48(1):21–9.

48. Hong JP. The use of super microsurgery in lower extremity reconstruction: the next step in evolution. Plast Reconstr Surg 2009;123(1):230–5.

49. Munhoz AM, Ishida LH, Montag E, et al. Perforator flap breast reconstruction using internal mammary perforator branches as a recipient site: an anatomical and clinical analysis. Plast Reconstr Surg 2004;114(1):62–8.

50. Haywood RM, Raurell A, Perks AG, et al. Autologous free tissue breast reconstruction using the internal mammary perforators as recipient vessels. Br J Plast Surg 2003;56(7):689–91.

51. Bayramiçli M, Yilmaz B, San T, et al. Effects of hematoma on the short-term fate of experimental microvenous autografts. J Reconstr Microsurg 1998;14(8): 575–86.

52. Li X, Cooley BC, Gould JS. Influence of topical heparin on stasis-induced thrombosis of microvascular anastomoses. Microsurgery 1992;13(2): 72–5.

53. Rumbolo PM, Cooley BC, Hanel DP, et al. Comparison of the influence of intralumenal irrigation solutions on free flap survival. Microsurgery 1992; 13(1):45–7.

54. Futran ND, Stack BC Jr. Single versus dual venous drainage of the radial forearm free flap. Am J Otolaryngol 1996;17(2):112–7.

55. Blackwell KE, Brown MT, Gonzalez D. Overcoming the learning curve in microvascular head and neck reconstruction. Arch Otolaryngol Head Neck Surg 1997;123(12):1332–5.

56. Blondeel P, Neligan PC. Complications: avoidance and treatment. In: Blondeel PN, Morris SF, Hallock GG, et al, editors. Perforator flaps: anatomy, technique & clinical applications. St Louis (MO): Quality Medical Pub; 2005. p. 116–28.

57. Kaplan JL, Allen RJ. Cost-based comparison between perforator flaps and TRAM flaps for breast reconstruction. Plast Reconstr Surg 2000;105(3): 943–8.

58. Serletti JM, Moran SL, Orlando GS, et al. Urokinase protocol for free-flap salvage following prolonged venous thrombosis. Plast Reconstr Surg 1998; 102(6):1947–53.

59. Panchapakesan V, Addison P, Beausang E, et al. Role of thrombolysis in free-flap salvage. J Reconstr Microsurg 2003;19(8):523–30.

60. Yii NW, Evans GR, Miller MJ, et al. Thrombolytic therapy: what is its role in free flap salvage? Ann Plast Surg 2001;46(6):601–4.

61. Wang WZ, Tsai TM, Anderson GL. Late-preconditioning protection is evident in the microcirculation of denervated skeletal muscle. J Orthop Res 1999; 17(4):571–7.

62. Bhat S, Shah A, Burd A. The role of freestyle perforator-based pedicled flaps in reconstruction of delayed traumatic defects. Ann Plast Surg 2009; 63(1):45–52.

63. Adler N, Dorafshar AH, Agarwal JP, et al. Harvesting the lateral femoral circumflex chimera free flap: guidelines for elevation. Plast Reconstr Surg 2009; 123(3):918–25.

The Integration of Muscle Perforator Flaps into a Community-Based Private Practice

Geoffrey G. Hallock, MD[a,b,c,]*

KEYWORDS

• Muscle perforator flap • Private practice • Microsurgery

In early 1984, Song and colleagues[1] showed how a large, undelayed fasciocutaneous flap could be reliably raised from the anterolateral thigh based on a septocutaneous perforator from the descending branch of the lateral circumflex femoral vessels. The author's senior partner at the time coincidentally was referred a patient who had degloved his ankle and heel pad in a motorcycle accident, with exposure of the Achilles tendon and multiple open fractures of the hindfoot (**Fig. 1**). Because of the extremely large size of the defect, he suggested that, although a novel idea, this thigh flap would be a terrific solution if used as a microsurgical transfer. The requisite huge flap was designed and raised following all of the instructions carefully; and predictably—in retrospect—no septocutaneous perforator could be found, but instead after dissection of the entire anterior thigh there was only a single, and what was considered a relatively tiny, musculocutaneous perforator of the vastus lateralis muscle. With no guidelines to follow, instead of abandoning this donor site, it seemed plausible to tediously dissect the perforator through the muscle, with careful coagulation of all muscular side branches, back to a reasonably large caliber source vessel. Despite the trepidation in doing this, the flap survived completely without further sequelae (see **Fig. 1**).

After gleaning through the original Song and colleagues[1] article now numerous times since, a fine print disclaimer is noted that states that occasionally the perforator to what is still today called the anterolateral thigh flap may pass "through a thin layer of muscle fibers before entering the skin."[1] The author's group had actually harvested a muscle perforator free flap without knowing it, because this appellation did not exist at that time. Compared with the more conventional muscle free flap donor sites in use then, this dissection had been so difficult and the stress of performing just a microvascular anastomosis was so great because the authors had just begun that learning curve that they vowed never to use this flap again. Little did they know what the future would bring.

Disregarding the preceding historical footnote, the role of fasciocutaneous flaps as a soft tissue alternative or supplement to muscle flaps, which were popular at that time, became obvious and otherwise intriguing.[2] A relatively obscure treatise in 1986 by Nakajima and colleagues[3] suggested that the deep fascia has 6 different types of perforators, and that each could potentially nourish a skin flap (**Fig. 2**). Although one of these, the *perforating cutaneous branch of muscular vessel*,[3] traversed the muscle, its intended course was primarily directly to the integument. They

a Division of Plastic Surgery, Sacred Heart Hospital, Allentown, PA, USA
b Division of Plastic Surgery, The Lehigh Valley Hospitals, Allentown, PA, USA
c Division of Plastic Surgery, St Luke's Hospital, Bethlehem, PA, USA
* 1230 South Cedar Crest Boulevard, Suite 306, Allentown, PA 18103.
E-mail address: pbhallock@cs.com

Clin Plastic Surg 37 (2010) 607–614
doi:10.1016/j.cps.2010.06.001
0094-1298/10/$ – see front matter © 2010 Elsevier Inc. All rights reserved.

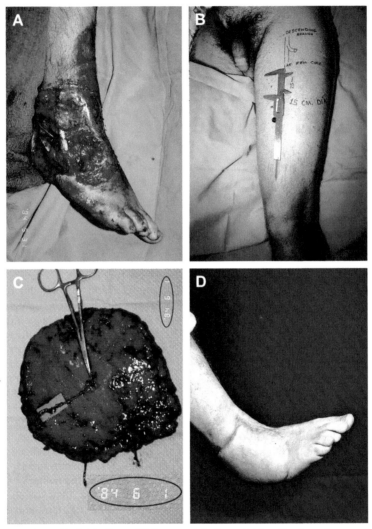

Fig. 1. (*A*) Degloving injury of left hindfoot. (*B*) Proposed design of thigh flap based on septocutaneous perforator presumed to be found at the junction of the middle and upper thirds of the thigh according to the instructions of Song and colleagues.[1] (*C*) Undersurface of free anterolateral thigh flap with what proved to be a musculocutaneous perforator (on microgrid) entering its center; note encircled date of event that is magnified in inset below. (*D*) Well-healed muscle perforator flap 1 year later that salvaged foot.

postulated that this perforator could stand alone to serve a "perforating cutaneous branch of muscular vessel flap."[3] Because this type of flap will always require the tedious intramuscular dissection of that musculocutaneous perforator, Wei and colleagues[4] defined these as "true" muscle perforator flaps.

The author's personal reindoctrination into this concept of muscle perforator flaps awaited his response to a flyer advertising the 5th International Course on Perforator Flaps in Gent, Belgium in 2001, at which Steve Morris had also matriculated to be an observer. As overseen by the course chairman, Philip Blondeel, the attributes of muscle perforator flaps became more apparent, including

their large potential size, large-caliber vessels with long vascular pedicles, and abundance of donor sites to better match the characteristics of any possible recipient site. In an attempt to be intimately involved in this nascent field, the author presented an abstract reviewing anatomic dissections of gastrocnemius musculocutaneous perforators[5] just before a clinical series by Cavadas and colleagues,[6] which is now known as the *sural artery perforator flap* according to the Canadian nomenclature terminology.[7] One of the panelists, Fu Chan Wei, in response to the author's question, actually entered the audience to debate just what were "perforator flaps." This discussion led to the idea that perforators could be "direct" or

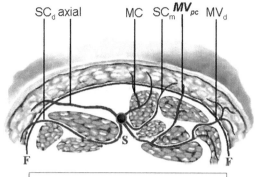

SC$_d$ axial   MC SC$_m$ *MV$_{pc}$* MV$_d$

axial = direct cutaneous
MC = musculocutaneous
MV$_d$ = direct cutaneous branch of
         muscular vessel
MV$_{pc}$= *perforating cutaneous branch*
         of muscular vessel
SC$_d$ = direct septocutaneous
SC$_m$ = minor septocutaneous

Fig. 2. Six different forms of perforators potentially pierce the deep fascia before proceeding to the integument, as listed.[3] Their "perforating cutaneous branch of muscular vessel" first traverses the given muscle with its destination primarily to be the overlying skin, to serve as the vascular pedicle of what today would be considered a "true" muscle perforator flap.[4] F, deep fascia; S, source vessel.

"indirect," with muscle perforator flaps the quintessential representative of the latter[8] and enduring as the primary topic of that course, and for the remainder of this compendium, for the sake of clarity.

METHOD AND MATERIALS

The author's private practice in a community setting started after completion of typical University training in 1982. Random flaps were still in vogue, and therefore this opportunity permitted the introduction of the relatively new concept of muscle flaps, followed soon after by various forms of fasciocutaneous flaps, both proving to be a better technique for soft tissue reconstruction (**Table 1**). Although readily transferred as local or pedicled flaps, the existing vacuum of other plausible alternatives allowed investigators to hone their microsurgical skills and enabled the simultaneous introduction of microvascular tissue transfers, or free flaps (see **Table 1**). From an awkward beginning, and thereafter often following a rocky road virtually without knowledgeable supervision, muscle perforator flaps were eventually reintegrated in 2001 (see **Table 1; Table 2**) into what has primarily been a solo practice within this same community from 1982 to now.

RESULTS

In the early 1980s, when a soft tissue reconstruction was considered by the author's group, muscle flaps were the predominant selection (see **Table 1**). By the 1990s, fasciocutaneous flaps had assumed an almost equivalent role, especially as a local flap option. Beginning in 2002, following the course in Gent, Belgium, muscle perforator flaps gradually assumed a role, primarily as a source of free tissue

Table 1
Timeline of the diversity of soft tissue flaps options used in the community setting[a]

| Year | Muscle | | Fasciocutaneous | | | |
| | | | Perforator | | Nonperforator | |
	Local Flap	Free Flap	Local Flap	Free Flap	Local Flap	Free Flap
1982–1986[b]	18	6			7	4
1987–1991[b]	13	8			21	5
1992–1996[b]	18	10			14	5
1997–2001[b]	32	18			13	4
2002	27	25	11	19	14	5
2003	34	30	5	6	14	4
2004	29	21	8	21	13	7
2005	38	16	8	29	13	3
2006	18	5	10	28	19	6
2007	18	10	11	27	16	4
2008	21	20	7	39	18	6

[a] From 1982 to 2008.
[b] Annual mean.

Table 2
Hierarchy of muscle perforator flap donor sites used in the community setting[a]

	Local Flap	Free Flap	Total
Anterolateral thigh	7	108	115
DIEP	3	29	32
SAP	16	15	31
MCFAP	7	19	26
GAP	13	1	14
All others	20	10	30
	66	182	248

Abbreviations: DIEP, deep inferior epigastric perforator; GAP, gluteal artery perforator; MCFAP, medial circumflex femoral artery perforator; SAP, sural artery perforator.
  [a] From 1984–2009 to date.

transfers. Although the frequency of muscle flap use has since diminished, the absolute number has remained relatively constant, reflecting the significant growth in the annual number of total flaps used as this practice matured, and the fact that use of muscle as a flap, despite prejudices otherwise, still has a viable role.[9]

The use of microsurgical tissue transfers has also increased dramatically in the past 5 years, and this seems to be the author's unadvertised niche in the Northeastern Pennsylvania region, with muscle perforator flaps far outperforming the numbers of muscle and other fasciocutaneous flaps combined (see **Table 1**).

Although many consider the "big four"[10] of muscle perforator flaps to be the anterolateral thigh flap (ALT), deep inferior epigastric perforator flap (DIEP), superior gluteal artery perforator flap (SGAP), and thoracodorsal artery perforator flap (TAP), the sural (SAP) and medial circumflex femoral artery perforator (MCFAP) flaps were more often selected by the author's group than the SGAP and TAP (see **Table 2**). The ALT flap certainly has been the most versatile donor site, providing large flaps with a relatively consistent anatomy and allowing a long pedicle of large caliber to reach recipient vessels outside the zone of injury with often "macrosurgical" anastomoses,[11] proving to be an ideal soft tissue flap.[12]

The DIEP flap has been the major source for autogenous tissue breast reconstruction in the author's practice, with this choice often being sought by patients who want to minimize any donor site morbidity.[13] In this group's experience, the MCFAP flap has been an excellent free tissue donor site in thinner individuals, whenever the ability to hide the donor site scar is of paramount importance.[14] Also known as the *medial groin flap*,[15,16] the resulting scar is easily hidden

completely by clothing. The SAP flaps are the source of a relatively thin cutaneous free flap, even in the most obese individual, that can be harvested with the patient in a supine or prone position.[17] Its greatest attribute has been its use as a local flap for knee coverage,[18] preserving gastrocnemius muscle function or holding it in reserve for later use.[19]

DISCUSSION

The evolution of the flap selection process in this community private practice, as used to solve the usual gamut of reconstructive challenges, has recapitulated the timeline of the general plastic surgery community. In the early 1980s, muscle flaps predominated as the preferred soft tissue flap, until Pontén's[20] "superflaps" reintroduced what would become the concept of a fascial plexus and the basis of fasciocutaneous flaps. Nakajima and colleagues[3] then theorized a subtype of fasciocutaneous flaps that would become the muscle perforator flap. Kroll and Rosenfield[21] introduced this as a clinical entity, but Koshima and Soeda[22] really deserve the credit for establishing this variant as an important alternative.

As long as a reasonable perforator can be found, a muscle perforator flap can be designed anywhere in the body, either as a local flap to bring similar characteristics in kind to an adjacent defect, or for identical reasons as a free flap to best match a recipient site elsewhere (see **Table 1**). It is ironic that the anterolateral thigh flap, so awkwardly first encountered in the author's initial experience (see **Fig. 1**), continues worldwide to be the most common donor site for a muscle perforator flap.[12] Its large size, reasonable anatomic consistency,[23] large caliber and long vascular leash, and possibility for numerous chimeric combinations[24] makes this the gold standard of muscle perforator flaps.

As is true for any new facet of life, there is a learning curve.[25] The same microsurgical skills essential for the successful transfer of a free flap will enable an almost innate, meticulous performance of the sometimes demanding dissection of diminutive musculocutaneous perforators; and possession of those skills will make this curve shorter. The author's group has been most fortunate that they have a microscope in their inner-city community hospital to facilitate this dissection whenever necessary. However, no particular new equipment is necessary, just the reasonable and steady hands of a dedicated surgeon willing to innovate a little. Because the author's facility is not as busy as its suburban hospital counterparts, more operative theater time has been allotted to clinicians in the practice to allow the requisite dissection of muscle perforator flaps in relative anonymity, which is important because these take a little longer than traditional flaps.

The limited resources of a community hospital require the author's group to anticipate some common pitfalls and concerns with muscle perforator flaps to minimize risks and complications. Anatomic anomalies are so common that these should be expected, in contradistinction to what the group thought was a misadventure during their original experience in 1984, described earlier. The advent of CT and MRI can facilitate the preoperative identification of requisite perforators[26–28] and may eventually eliminate any exploratory guesswork, but these tests are expensive and not without risk, and therefore the author's group still relies on the traditional acoustic Doppler ultrasound despite its shortcomings, because it is readily available even in the poorest hospital.[29]

Despite sophisticated three- and four-dimensional perfusion studies intended to document the anatomic and perhaps dynamic territory of a given perforator,[30,31] an uncertainty persists because of the great variability among individuals. Therefore, whenever possible to theoretically enhance flap perfusion, the author's group preserves dual perforators that are preferably at opposite extremes of the chosen flap (**Fig. 3**). Another advantage of this configuration is that it will be virtually impossible to accidentally twist and compromise the vascular pedicle, and it also serves as an added safety factor in case of inadvertent injury to one perforator that would otherwise condemn the flap to certain failure. Unfortunately, sometimes this results in a vascular pedicle that is exceedingly long (yet sometimes also an attribute of muscle perforator flaps), and could be subject to kinking unless the surgeon is very careful (see **Fig. 3**).

Venous congestion is another potential problem associated with muscle perforator flaps, because venous outflow does not always follow the same course as the arterial inflow.[32] Again, whenever possible, a subcutaneous vein is preserved as an alternative outflow tract to allow later venous supercharging if indicated. This technique is a recognized solution for the DIEP flap, with retention of a sizeable superficial inferior epigastric vein, if encountered, considered mandatory (**Fig. 4**).[33]

Another frequent cause of venous congestion is excessive pressure on the low-pressure venous

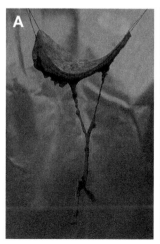
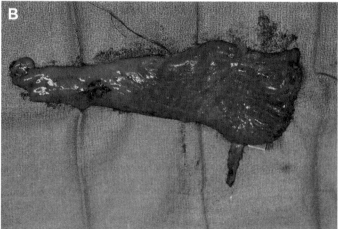

Fig. 3. (A) Dual perforators arising from the same source vessel in this anterolateral thigh free flap were both retained because they were similar in size and reasonably separated from each other to theoretically more reliably capture a greater territory. Note the extremely long vascular leash that is possible (B), especially when compared with that of the gracilis muscle, which has a notoriously short pedicle.

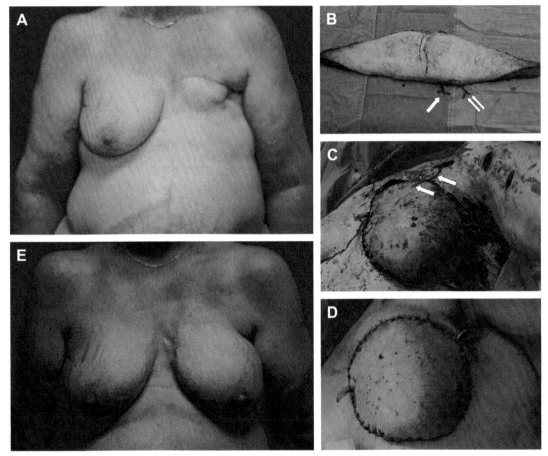

Fig. 4. (*A*) Preoperative candidate who desired autogenous tissues for left breast reconstruction. (*B*) Harvested deep inferior epigastric perforator flap showing the major deep inferior epigastric pedicle (*arrow*), and lateral to it the retained superficial inferior epigastric vein (SIEV; *double arrow*). (*C*) The internal mammary vessels served as the recipient site, but venous congestion ensued. The left cephalic vein (*arrows*) was harvested from the arm through small incisions and coupled to the SIEV to supercharge venous outflow from the flap, with immediate resolution of congestion (*D*), and a reasonable result after nipple creation and areolar micropigmentation (*E*).

side after the "perfect" inset, which may not manifest until after the usual postoperative flap edema occurs. This event can be avoided altogether by leaving the subcutaneous tissues on one boundary of the flap untethered and exposed (**Fig. 5**); eventually this side will close spontaneously through the natural process of wound contraction.

SUMMARY

The integration of muscle perforator flaps into the author's reconstructive practice has been a natural and positive experience, allowing greater diversity in flap selection to be offered to the patient population. The problems are no different in patients who present to a community hospital. The author has had the good fortune to be a recipient of Philip Blondeel's zeal in spreading the "gospel" of perforator flaps, and the intellectual stimulus of

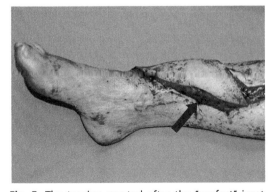

Fig. 5. The tension created after the "perfect" inset, especially when closing a thick muscle perforator flap, can potentially impede venous outflow. This event can be minimized by closing only the deeper subcutaneous tissue layer of the flap to the defect (*arrow*) to avoid excessive pressure.

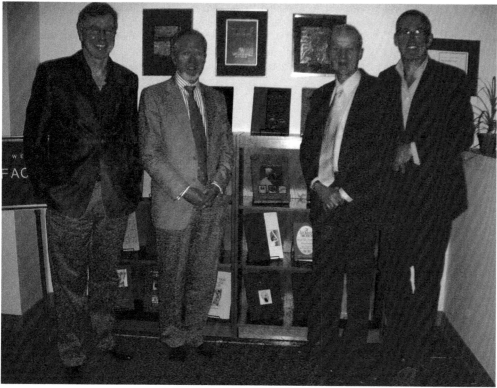

Fig. 6. The "Perforator Gang of Four"—Steve Morris, Peter Neligan, Geoff Hallock, and Phillip Blondeel, (*left* to *right*)—networking in the library.

continuing debates over small details such as nomenclature. The author's colleagues Steve Morris and Peter Neligan have tried to solve this dilemma with their Canadian system.[7] This collaboration has improved global communication and the disbursement of constant improvements in this dynamic field wherever needed (**Fig. 6**), whether now virtually instantaneously through the Internet or still with the written word.[34] Supermicrosurgery, as spearheaded by Koshima and colleagues,[35] may someday allow futuristic "capillary" perforator flaps even to be a mainstay of the community hospital. Time will tell the pathway the field will follow.

ACKNOWLEDGMENTS

Alan E. Trevaskis, MD, was my original senior partner who recognized the future role of microsurgery in reconstructive surgery even in the community setting, and by serendipity introduced me to what would become "muscle perforator flaps." David C. Rice, BS, recognized in this text whenever the plural nominative case was used, helped us develop de novo the microsurgical expertise necessary for microvascular anastomoses, and

the related techniques required for the proper harvest of muscle perforator flaps.

REFERENCES

1. Song TG, Chen GZ, Song YL. The free thigh flap: a new free flap concept based on the septocutaneous artery. Br J Plast Surg 1984;37:149-59.
2. Hallock GG. Fasciocutaneous flaps. Cambridge (MA): Blackwell Scientific Publications; 1992.
3. Nakajima H, Fujino T, Adachi S. A new concept of vascular supply to the skin and classification of skin flaps according to their vascularization. Ann Plast Surg 1986;16:1-17.
4. Wei FC, Jain V, Suominen S, et al. Confusion among perforator flaps: what is a true perforator flap? Plast Reconstr Surg 2001;107:874-6.
5. Hallock GG. Anatomic basis of the gastrocnemius perforator-based flap. Ann Plast Surg 2001;47:517-22.
6. Cavadas PC, Sanz-Gimenez-Rico JR, Gutierrez-de la Camara A, et al. The medial sural artery perforator free flap. Plast Reconstr Surg 2001;108:1609-15.
7. Geddes CR, Morris SF, Neligan PC. Perforator flaps: evolution, classification, and applications. Ann Plast Surg 2003;50:90-9.

8. Hallock GG. Direct and indirect perforator flaps: the history and the controversy. Plast Reconstr Surg 2003;111:855–66.

9. Hallock GG. In an era of perforator flaps, are muscle flaps passé? Plast Reconstr Surg 2009; 123:1357–63.

10. Hallock GG. A primer of schematics to facilitate the design of the preferred muscle perforator flaps. Plast Reconstr Surg 2009;123:1107–15.

11. Hallock GG. Macrovascular surgery and the microsurgeon. J Reconstr Microsurg 1997;13:563–9.

12. Wei FC, Jain V, Celik N, et al. Have we found an ideal soft-tissue flap? an experience with 672 anterolateral thigh flaps. Plast Reconstr Surg 2002;109:2219–26.

13. Blondell PN, Vanderstraeten GG, Monstrey SJ, et al. The donor site morbidity of free DIEP flaps and free TRAM flaps for breast reconstruction. Br J Plast Surg 1997;50:322–30.

14. Hallock GG. The development of the medial circumflex femoral artery perforator (MCFAP) flap. Sem Plast Surg 2006;20:121–6.

15. Hallock GG. The medial circumflex femoral GRACILIS local perforator flap–a local medial groin perforator flap. Ann Plast Surg 2003;51:460–4.

16. Hallock GG. The gracilis (medial circumflex femoral) perforator flap: a medial groin free flap? Ann Plast Surg 2003;51:623–6.

17. Hallock GG, Sano K. The medial sural medial gastrocnemius perforator free flap: an "ideal" prone position skin flap. Ann Plast Surg 2004;52:184–7.

18. Hallock GG. The medial sural medial gastrocnemius perforator local flap. Ann Plast Surg 2004;53:501–5.

19. Hallock GG. Sequential use of a true perforator flap and its corresponding muscle flap. Ann Plast Surg 2003;51:617–20.

20. Pontén B. The fasciocutaneous flap: its use in soft tissue defects of the lower leg. Br J Plast Surg 1981;34:215–20.

21. Kroll SS, Rosenfield L. Perforator-based flaps for low posterior midline defects. Plast Reconstr Surg 1988; 81:561–6.

22. Koshima I, Soeda S. Inferior epigastric artery skin flaps without rectus abdominis muscle. Br J Plast Surg 1989;42:645–8.

23. Yu P, Youssef A. Efficacy of the handheld Doppler in preoperative identification of the cutaneous perforators in the anterolateral thigh flap. Plast Reconstr Surg 2006;118:928–33.

24. Wei FC, Celik N, Jeng SF. Application of "simplified nomenclature for compound flaps" to the anterolateral thigh flap. Plast Reconstr Surg 2005;115: 1051–5.

25. Hallock GG. Is there a "learning curve" for muscle perforator flaps? Ann Plast Surg 2008;60:146–9.

26. Masiá J, Larrañaga J, Clavero JA, et al. The value of the multidetector row computed tomography for the preoperative planning of deep inferior epigastric artery perforator flap, our experience in 162 cases. Ann Plast Surg 2008;60:29–36.

27. Rozen WM, Phillips TJ, Ashton MW, et al. Preoperative imaging for DIEP perforator flaps: a comparative study of computed tomographic angiography and Doppler ultrasound. Plast Reconstr Surg 2008;121: 9–16.

28. de Weerd L, Weum S, Mercer JB. The value of dynamic infrared thermography (DIRT) in perforator selection and planning of free DIEP flaps. Ann Plast Surg 2009;63:274–9.

29. Hallock GG. Attributes and shortcomings of acoustic Doppler sonography in identifying perforators for flaps from the lower extremity. J Reconstr Microsurg 2009;25:377–82.

30. Saint-Cyr M, Schaverien M, Arbique G, et al. Three- and four-dimensional computed tomographic angiography and venography for the investigation of the vascular anatomy and perfusion of perforator flaps. Plast Reconstr Surg 2008;121:772–80.

31. Schaverien M, Saint-Cyr M, Arbique G, et al. Three- and four-dimensional computed topographic angiography and venography of the anterolateral thigh perforator flap. Plast Reconstr Surg 2008;121: 1685–96.

32. Schaverien M, Saint-Cyr M, Arbique G, et al. Anatomies of the deep inferior epigastric perforator and superficial inferior epigastric artery flaps. Plast Reconstr Surg 2008;1221:1909–19.

33. Villafane O, Gahankari D, Webster M. Superficial inferior epigastric vein (SIEV): lifeboat for DIEP/TRAM flaps [letter]. Br J Plast Surg 1999;52:599.

34. Blondeel PN, Morris SF, Hallock GG, et al. Perforator flaps: anatomy, technique, clinical applications. St. Louis (MO): Quality Medical Publishing; 2006.

35. Koshima I, Nanba Y, Takahasi Y, et al. Future of supramicrosurgery as it relates to breast reconstruction: free paraumbilical perforator adiposal flap. Sem Plast Surg 2002;16:93–9.

The Propeller Flap Concept

Tiew Chong Teo, MD (Hons), FRCS (Plast)

KEYWORDS

- Propeller flap • Perforator flap • Local flap
- Lower limb reconstruction • Free flap • Microsurgery

EVOLUTION

Wounds on the distal third of the lower extremity are known to be difficult to reconstruct. The lack of spare local tissue in the immediate vicinity of such wounds makes it difficult to design local flaps. With unreliable outcomes and increased morbidity, the general perception is that a free flap is the preferred option. However, I have always found it difficult to accept that a small to medium-sized defect on the distal third of the lower leg can only be reliably covered by a free flap.

In the 1980s, Ponten[1] and Barclay and colleagues[2] published the first clinical reports on fasciocutaneous flaps showing that long flaps can safely stretch the length to width ratio of random pattern flaps from 1:1 to 3:1. Their results generated much interest and stimulated many studies into peripheral vascularization of the skin through perforators.[3–5] Surgeons who realized the importance of perforators began to preserve the myocutaneous or septocutaneous perforators when designing new flaps. Donski and Fogdestam[6] demonstrated that such long flaps could just as safely be based distally on the lower peroneal perforators and used for reconstruction of defects around the lower third of the leg. These investigators postulated that by keeping the long axis of the flap on top of the posterior peroneal intermuscular septum, the perforators linked within the flap, forming an "axial pattern" blood flow that was therefore able to sustain a longer flap than would otherwise be possible. Amarante and colleagues[7] showed that the lower posterior tibial artery perforators could equally be used safely to base such peninsular fasciocutaneous flaps for covering defects around the lower third of the leg. Gradually, the design of the skin bridge at the base of such peninsular flaps was being made progressively narrower until some surgeons felt brave enough to totally divide it and completely island the flaps. These investigators realized that keeping the skin bridge at the base of a peninsular flap does not improve its blood supply and may in fact kink the pedicle, contributing to vascular embarrassment of the flap. Furthermore, it was evident that the bulky "dog ear" was visually unappealing.[8,9] These surgeons were also the first to routinely visualize the perforators and eventually isolate the flap on to a single perforator, but they remained reluctant to handle or clean around the pedicle.[10] Most reports were of very few cases until Erdmann and colleagues[10] reported the first big series from which they concluded that the distally based islanded fasciocutaneous flap was a good first choice for coverage of defects on the lower third of the leg and ankle.

WHAT IS THE PROPELLER FLAP?

The propeller flap is a local island fasciocutaneous flap based on a single dissected perforator. It is designed like a propeller with 2 blades of unequal length with the perforator forming the pivot point so that when the blades are switched, the long arm comfortably fills in the defect (**Fig. 1**). The ability of this flap to rotate any angle up to 180° makes it extremely versatile for reconstructing traumatic as well as other defects of the distal lower limb where it was originally conceived. Gradually its use has been extended for reconstruction of many defects of varying etiology throughout the

Department of Plastic Surgery, Queen Victoria Hospital, Holtye Road, East Grinstead, West Sussex RH19 3DZ, UK
E-mail address: tc.teo@qvh.nhs.uk

Clin Plastic Surg 37 (2010) 615–626
doi:10.1016/j.cps.2010.06.003
0094-1298/10/$ – see front matter © 2010 Published by Elsevier Inc.

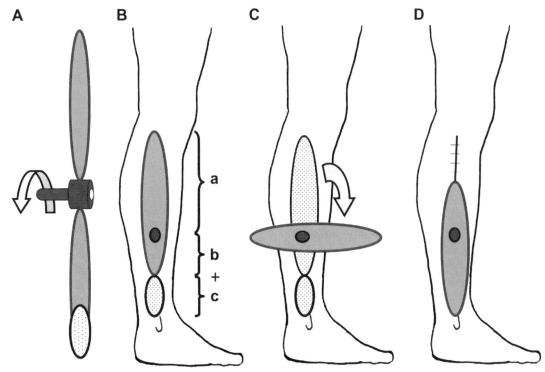

Fig. 1. (*A*) The propeller flap concept can be thought of as a propeller with 2 blades of unequal length with the perforator forming the pivot point; when the blades are switched, the long arm comfortably fills in the defect. (*B*) Marking of the flap. The distance between the perforator and the proximal tip of the flap (a) is equal to length of the defect (c) plus the distance between the proximal edge of the defect and the perforator (b) with 1 cm added to allow for the tissue retraction and to facilitate tension free closure when the flap is rotated. The width of the flap is equal to the width of the defect with 0.5 cm added. (*C*) After the flap and the perforator are completely dissected, the flap is rotated to cover the defect. (*D*) The short arm of the propeller flap is used to aid closure of the secondary defect either completely or with a skin graft.

body. The propeller flap concept is best explained by addressing 3 key questions.

Why Does it have to be Based Distally for the Distal Lower Limb Reconstruction?

The lower leg is shaped like a cone tapering down toward the lower third and ankle with a paucity of spare tissue in that area for use in reconstructing defects. For this reason a proximally based peninsular fasciocutaneous flap tends to struggle in terms of getting enough healthy tissue into the defect and, in addition, it risks exposing either the subcutaneous border of the tibia or the Achilles tendon, both of which are difficult to graft and could often be prone to unstable scarring in the long term. The propeller flap, pivoted on a single perforator, avoids these problems by importing truly undamaged tissue from the proximal calf into the primary defect. In doing so it simultaneously transfers the secondary defect to an easily graftable area over the proximal muscle bellies. Even better, when there is tissue laxity in the

proximal calf, the propeller flap can often allow the secondary defect to be closed primarily.

Why Does it have to be Based on only a Single Pedicle?

A logical question, because if one perforator is safe surely two should be safer. However, the design of this flap makes the use of more than one pedicle a potential hazard because the two pedicles could kink each other (**Fig. 2**) or, in trying to avoid this problem, the rotation of the flap becomes limited. When the rotation is needed only up to 90° it may not matter if more than one pedicle is kept. However, when the flap is needed to rotate 180° it is actually safer to divide all perforators except one.

Why Island the Flap?

This is also a safety issue because the skin connection of a peninsular flap makes an awkward and unsightly twist at its base, which could risk compressing and stretching the pedicle and

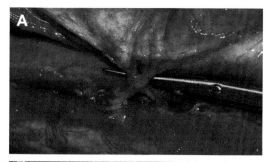

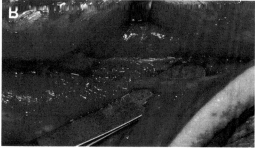

Fig. 2. (*A, B*) The propeller flap should not be based on 2 perforators because, with the rotation of the flap, the 2 pedicles are twisted around each other and this can jeopardize its blood supply. Basing the flap on a single pedicle is safer and it also facilitates flap rotation and inset.

potentially cause the flap to suffer. In contrast, the cutting of all the soft tissue connections to truly island the propeller flap gives it a much greater freedom to pivot and rotate around its pedicle. This procedure also allows for a more distal reach of the flap on to the dorsum and lateral aspect of the foot when needed. It is also easier to inset and gives a better final contour.

SURGICAL TECHNIQUE
Propeller Flap for Distal Lower Limb Defects

Guidelines
In the lower limb, the main useful perforators arise from the 3 major vessels—the posterior tibial, the peroneal, and the anterior tibial arteries. In my experience, it is easier to base the flap on the perforators arising from the first 2 vessels. As mentioned before, in designing the flap it is best to avoid transgressing onto the subcutaneous border of the tibia as well as the Achilles tendon. Also, it would be desirable to try to avoid damage to the saphenous nerve or the sural nerve depending on which side of the leg the flap is based.

It is important to adopt a flexible approach in the design and execution of the procedure, and although this may sound daunting to the beginner, following a few simple rules makes it a straightforward operation.

Design of the flap
Preoperatively, a handheld 8- to 10-MHz Doppler ultrasound scanner is helpful to locate the most promising perforator artery near the defect. A provisional flap design can then be drawn as follows, with the perforator as the pivot point of the flap (**Fig. 3**A). First, the distance between the perforator and the distal edge of the defect is measured. This value is then transposed proximally along the axis of the main source vessel, again measured from the perforator, and 1 cm is added. This value forms the proximal limit of the flap. Next, the width of the proximal flap needed to cover the defect is determined by measuring the width of the defect. This value is then used to determine the proximal flap width, adding 0.5 cm to allow for flap contraction and to facilitate its inset without tension. It is also important to ensure that, at the pivot point where the perforator pedicle enters the flap, the lateral dimensions are equidistant to ensure that when the flap is eventually rotated around to fill the defect there is no excessive sideways traction on the perforator during wound closure.

Raising the flap
A thigh tourniquet is used, and the leg is exsanguinated by elevation and compression of the popliteal artery for 1 minute. This procedure allows emptying of most of the blood from the leg but retains enough in the perforator vessels to allow for easier identification during exploration.

The perforator vessels are located through an exploratory initial incision (**Fig. 3**B). It is important for safety and easier assessment to make this incision quite generous. The approach to the pedicle could be suprafascial or subfascial. Unless the surgeon is already experienced in raising perforator flaps, the subfascial approach is recommended as an easier and safer way to visualize the pedicle. With this initial incision, several potentially useful perforators are usually exposed and the best is chosen based on its position and size. In general, it would be wise to avoid any perforator that is encased in scar or granulation tissue near the edge of an acute or chronic wound because the dissection can prove difficult, with injury to an already fragile vessel more likely. On the other hand, it is best not to choose a perforator too far away from the defect, as this would make the flap unnecessarily long.

When the decision is made, the perforator that is finally chosen for the flap may not necessarily be the one located preoperatively on Doppler ultrasonography and on which the initial design of the flap is based. This is not a problem because the planning and initial steps in the raising of the flap allow

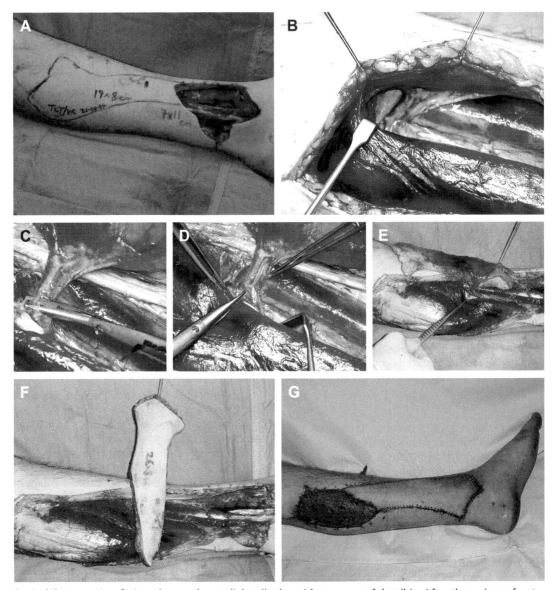

Fig. 3. (*A*) Traumatic soft tissue loss on the medial malleolus with exposure of the tibia. After the main perforator, arising from the posterior tibial artery, has been located with a handheld Doppler ultrasound scanner, the flap is planned around it. (*B*) A generous exploratory incision is made on the posterior border of the flap and the perforator on which the flap is based is visualized. (*C, D*) Meticulous dissection of the perforator. To avoid vascular compromise the perforator should be skeletonized completely by dividing all the fascial strands that could cause extrinsic compression, particularly of the venae comitantes, once the flap is rotated. (*E, F*) The flap, completely islanded on a single perforator, is then rotated to cover the defect. (*G*) Result at 1 month after surgery.

the surgeon the freedom to redesign and adjust its dimension, making it a flexible approach in raising the propeller flap. Once the best pedicle has been chosen, the design of the flap should be rechecked and, if necessary, adjusted. In particular, one should ensure that the proximal edge of the flap, when finally rotated into position, is capable of reaching the distal margin of the defect

comfortably and would not place the pedicle under any tension.

Once the critical decision is made about which perforator to use, time should then be spent in carefully preparing the pedicle. It should be cleared of all muscular side branches for at least 2 cm. This procedure allows a gentle spiral twist of the pedicle when the flap is rotated through

180°. When possible, the pedicle is cleaned from its source vessel to the point where it passes through the deep fascia into the flap. Next, all the fine fascial strands that could potentially compress the vessels once they are twisted should be meticulously divided (**Fig. 3**C, D). Particular attention should be paid to those around the venae comitantes, because the relatively low pressure venous system is more susceptible to extrinsic compression once the flap is rotated into position. Once the pedicle is secured, raising the rest of the flap is quick and straightforward. When the flap has been completely islanded, it should be left in its original position and the tourniquet is released (**Fig. 3**E). It is important to allow it to perfuse and the spasm of the vessels to relax for 10 to 15 minutes before the flap is rotated into the defect. Topical vasodilators, such as papaverine or verapamil, can be instilled around the pedicle at this point.

Rotation and inset of the flap

Once the flap perfusion is satisfactory, it is ready to be rotated into the defect (**Fig. 3**F). The flap is carefully lifted from the wound bed and pivoted around its pedicle. The direction of rotation depends on the angle between the proximal long axis of the flap and the defect. This angle can reach a maximum of 180°. It is not necessary to rotate the flap beyond 180° because it can simply be turned in the other direction. When the defect is at the 6 o'clock position and the flap has to be rotated 180°, the pedicle is placed under the maximum spiral twist. In this situation I always first turn the flap clockwise into the defect and, focusing on how comfortably the venae comitantes are positioned, look for any sign of extrinsic compression by residual fascial strands, which will need further division. I will then turn the flap counterclockwise and do the same examination of the pedicle. Once I decide which rotational direction is the most comfortable for the venae comitantes I then secure the flap into position with the first 2 skin sutures placed on either side of the axis of the pedicle. These 2 sutures should be carefully positioned to ensure that the pedicle is not put under any traction either in a proximal or distal direction. If a suction drain is used it should be placed and secured well away from pedicle. Thereafter the rest of the flap inset and wound closure should be straightforward. If the donor defect can be closed without excessive tension this, simplifies the final stages of the operation and produces the best aesthetic result. However, one should not be tempted to close the secondary defect of the wound so tightly as to jeopardize the blood supply of the flap or cause swelling of the distal leg from a tourniquet effect. In that situation a skin graft is preferable (**Fig. 3**G).

Indications

The propeller flap can be used to cover awkward defects on the distal third of the lower limb and around the ankle joint, including the medial and lateral malleoli,[11] which are common sites of poor healing following compound fractures and internal fixation (**Fig. 4**). Wound breakdown following repair of the Achilles tendon as well as an anterior wound problem complicating ankle arthroplasty could also be successfully addressed with the propeller flap. The flap can be extended to reach defects on the lateral border of the foot where wound dehiscence complicating internal fixation of calcaneal fractures are not uncommon.

For the middle and upper third of the leg and around the knee, the propeller flap can also be considered as an option, and a well-designed flap can allow direct closure of the secondary defect. The propeller flap produces a better contour by avoiding the dog-ear and bulkiness associated with the traditional proximally based peninsular fasciocutaneous flap and the medial gastrocnemius flap.

Propeller Flap for Upper Limb Defects

Guidelines

As in the lower extremity, the main perforators of the upper limb originate from the major arteries—brachial artery and profunda brachii in the upper arm, and radial, ulnar, anterior, and posterior interosseous arteries in the forearm. The perforators follow the intermuscular septa distally but proximally they often pierce the muscle bellies. In the upper arm they arise from the lateral septum between triceps and brachialis muscles and from the medial intermuscular septum between triceps and biceps. Around the elbow, the perforators arising from the brachial artery pierce the deep fascia on the medial and lateral sides of the biceps tendon. The perforators of the radial recurrent artery pierce the brachioradialis muscle. The perforators of the radial artery can be found proximally in the septum between the brachioradialis and pronator teres, and distally between the brachioradialis and flexor carpi radialis. The ulnar artery perforators arise in the septum between flexor carpi ulnaris and flexor digitorum superficialis.[12]

On the extensor aspect, the main perforators, arising from the posterior interosseous artery, emerge between the extensor carpi ulnaris and extensor digiti minimi in the upper two-thirds of the forearm. In the distal forearm the perforators derive from the dorsal branch of the anterior

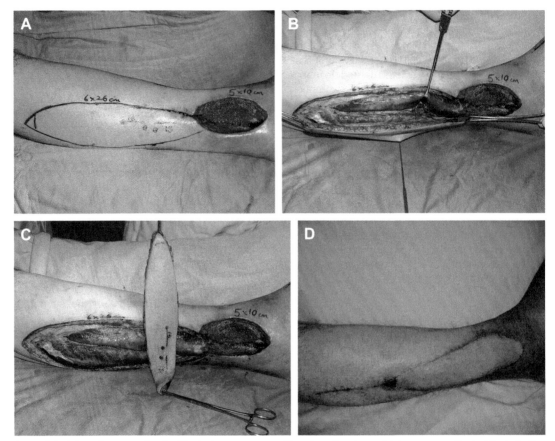

Fig. 4. (*A*) This patient sustained a fibula fracture treated by plate fixation, which was complicated by infection and wound breakdown. After removal of the plate and several debridements, a propeller flap based on a peroneal artery perforator was designed. (*B*) The exploratory incision allows the location and selection of the most suitable perforator, after which the flap is completely islanded. (*C, D*) The flap is rotated 180°, achieving coverage of the defect and primary closure of the proximal secondary defect with the result at 1 month.

interosseous artery, and they pass between extensor digitorum communis and extensor digiti minimi to reach the skin.[12]

This basic understanding of the possible location of the perforators is useful, especially in the distal forearm, where the radial and ulnar arteries are very superficial and Doppler ultrasonography is of limited use in differentiating source vessels from perforators.[13] Whenever possible, surgery should be performed using an arm tourniquet. The upper limb is elevated and the brachial artery is compressed for 1 minute to partially empty the vessels while retaining enough blood to facilitate the identification and dissection of the perforators. After the final size of the defect is determined, the nearby perforators can be explored subfascially either by lifting the margins of the wound or through an exploratory incision. The incision should be placed, depending on the location of the defect, on the volar or dorsal midlines or alternatively on the midlateral lines. Once the best

perforator is selected the flap can be designed and dissected as outlined in the previous section.

Indications

The propeller flap can be used for reconstruction of upper limb and hand defects following trauma, burns, and cancer resection. Because the upper extremity is often exposed, it is worth remembering that a good aesthetic outcome is just as important as a functional one; and an already injured hand certainly does not need further insult. Badly designed flaps, combined with extensive skin grafting, can produce a distressing result. The propeller flap can be selectively used for a good aesthetic outcome if it is designed in such a way that the secondary defect can be closed directly (**Fig. 5**). As in the lower limb, it can be used to bring proximal soft tissues into the distal defects of the forearm, wrist, and hand; and the avoidance of a dog-ear tends to produce a better contoured result. I find that one of the

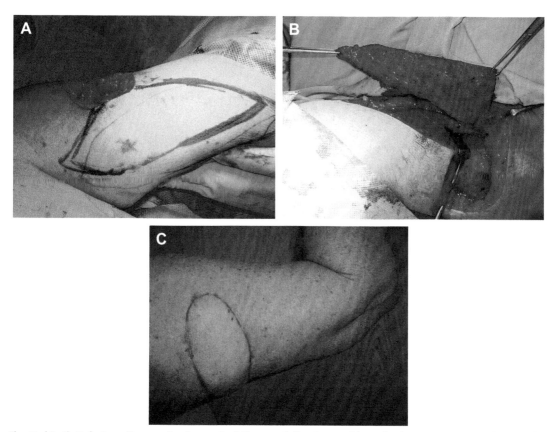

Fig. 5. (*A, B*) Defect on the proximal aspect of the arm following excision of a basosquamous carcinoma. The propeller flap is raised on a perforator arising from the profunda brachii artery and rotated 90° into the defect. (*C*) Final result at 6 months. The donor site was closed directly.

potential limitations to the wider application of the propeller flap in the distal forearm is the relatively short pedicle, which does not tend to withstand extreme (180°) rotation so well. One solution is, of course, to pedicle the flap on the radial or ulna artery, but the sacrifice of a major source vessel to the hand does give rise to concern.

Propeller Flap for Defects on the Trunk and Breast

Guidelines
When planning flaps on the anterior chest wall, it is important not to damage or distort the nipple areolar complex on the male chest and the breast in the female patient. The spare tissue tends to be found on the lateral chest wall above and below these structures. One should try, where possible, to place the scars within the subcostal and infra-mammary regions. The internal mammary artery perforators form 2 vertical rows exiting through the intercostal spaces about a finger's breadth

on either sides of the sternum. The other source of perforators is the acromiothoracic trunk that supplies the pectoral muscles. These perforators are suitable to base flaps for defects on the pre-sternal areas (**Fig. 6**). The upper ones can be used for flaps that will reach the lower neck while the lower ones, arising as anterior intercostal perforators from the musculophrenic artery (one of the terminal branches of the internal mammary artery) can be used to design flaps that will reach defects on the breast, epigastric, subcostal, and upper abdominal regions.

For the abdomen, the other terminal branch of the internal mammary artery, which becomes the superior epigastric artery, is the source of multiple perforators on which local perforator flaps can be based. For the lower half of the abdomen, the perforators arising from the inferior epigastric artery can be the basis for local flaps even though they are more commonly associated with the free deep inferior epigastric perforator flap. On the flank the terminal branches of the lumbar vessels

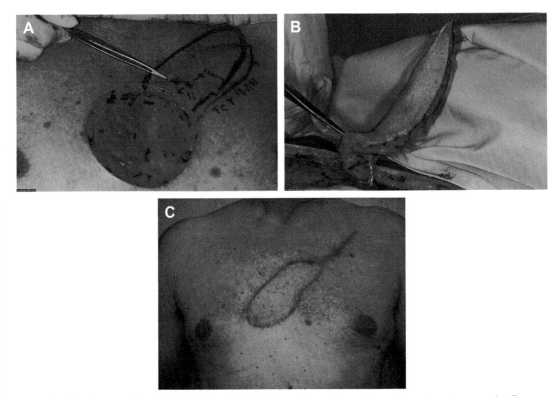

Fig. 6. (*A, B*) Defect on the anterior chest wall following wide excision of a malignant melanoma. The flap was planned and raised around an internal mammary artery perforator as indicated. (*C*) Final result with direct closure of the secondary defect achieving an excellent contour.

can be occasionally useful for basing lateral flaps, which can be turned in to reconstruct a central abdominal defect.

On the upper and mid back, the perforators that supply the skin arise from vessels that supply the underlying muscles such as the thoracodorsal for the latissimus dorsi muscle. The intercostal arteries also send several perforators through the intercostal spaces to supply the skin of the back. In this region, a search around the periphery of the defect to be reconstructed will usually yield several decent vessels for a sizeable flap to be raised.

In the lumbar region, 4 lumbar arteries arise from the aorta and pass laterally through the muscle layers of the posterior and lateral abdominal wall. These arteries can supply the perforators for flaps needed to cover defects on the back and flank. Flaps here are usually best designed transversely or obliquely to make use of the axiality of vessels. Here the closure of the secondary defect does not tend to be a problem because the flank area normally has good tissue laxity (**Fig. 7**).

Indications

On the anterior chest, propeller flaps can allow closure of defects to produce a more finely contoured result than would otherwise be achieved with a skin graft. Although not indicated for every patient, the aesthetic improvement that can be achieved makes it an option to consider (see **Fig. 6**). The anterior intercostal artery perforators can be used to base flaps, lying along the inframammary crease, which can be turned superiorly to cover defects on the medial aspect of the breast. The scar from the secondary defect closure is well hidden.

In the axillary region, the thoracodorsal artery and the posterior intercostal artery perforators are particularly useful for basing flaps that will import tissue from the back to reach defects on the lateral aspect of the breast.

Flaps are not often indicated on the abdomen because there is usually sufficient tissue to allow a direct closure of a wound. Occasionally, propeller flaps based on either the superior or inferior epigastric as well as the intercostal arteries can be designed to import healthy tissue into a defect scarred by multiple intra-abdominal procedures.

Propeller Flap for Defects on the Buttock

Guidelines

The superior and inferior gluteal arteries supply the skin through multiple myocutaneous perforators in

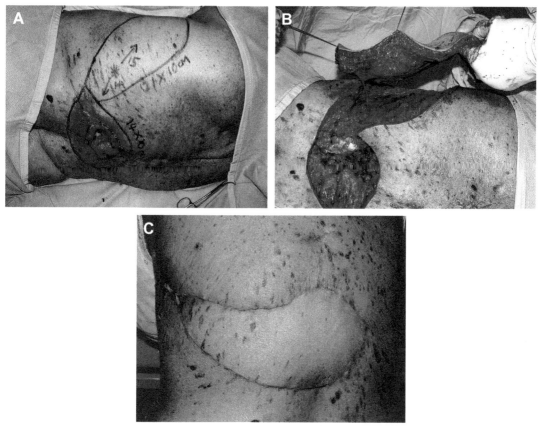

Fig. 7. (*A, B*) Large basal cell carcinoma on the back. After a wide local excision of the lesion, a 21 × 10-cm propeller flap, raised on an intercostal artery perforator, was used to cover the defect. (*C*) Result at 3 months' follow-up.

the buttock region, and this gives rise to multiple options in propeller flap planning. Following the radical excision of chronic infected wounds, including all the undermined and indurated areas, the resulting defect is usually quite sizeable. This defect may allow the location of perforators in the vicinity of the wound by lifting the skin edges around the defect. Alternatively, a generous exploratory incision is made on one edge of a pre-planned flap based on a perforator located by Doppler ultrasonography preoperatively. The skin is raised in the plane below the fascia overlying the muscle until the perforator is reached and confirmed to be suitable. The perforator is next dissected by widely splitting the muscle along the line of its fibers. It cannot be emphasized enough that the key to a safe dissection is to ensure that the muscle is split widely so that a decent length of perforator, about 3 to 4 cm, can be dissected out to allow a comfortable rotation of the flap. If the muscle appears to compress the pedicle then some of the fibers around it can safely be cut with no resultant functional loss.

The flap dimension is rechecked in relation to the position of the perforator before the flap is islanded and rotated into the defect. Usually an obliquely orientated flap would allow for easy closure of the secondary defect.

Indications

Propeller flaps used to reconstruct sacral and ischial (**Fig. 8**) pressure sore defects have proven to be robust and appear to withstand weight bearing well, even though they are not sensate flaps. Most of these flaps do develop some peripheral reinnervation, but the lack of full protective sensation does not lead to inevitable breakdown. Propeller flaps can also be used to resurface wounds in the trochanteric region derived from pressure ulceration or complications following orthopedic procedures.

Propeller flaps based on superior gluteal perforators are particularly successful for reconstructing defects following the radical resection of very scarred and infected pilonidal sinuses. The knowledge that one can import healthy tissue into the

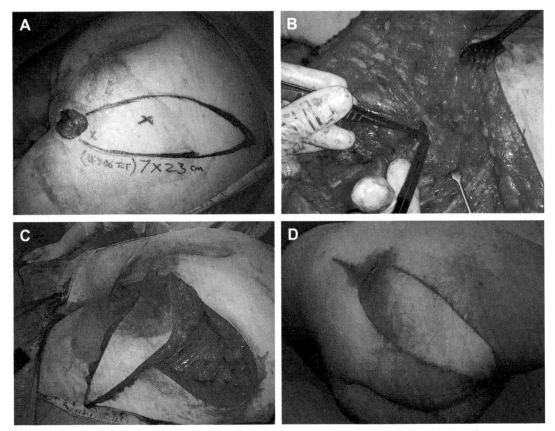

Fig. 8. (*A–C*) Following radical debridement of this ischial pressure sore, a propeller flap based on a superior gluteal artery perforator was raised and rotated 180° into the defect. (*D*) Durable result at 8 months after surgery.

defect for a tension-free closure allows the surgeon to radically resect all unhealthy infected and indurated tissue, which is the key to a successful outcome.

SAFETY AND RELIABILITY

Since 1992, when I performed my first propeller flap to cover a defect in the Achilles tendon region of the leg, more than 130 such flaps have been used to cover defects on the upper and lower limbs as well as the trunk. The indications included defects following trauma, cancer resection, chronic infection, pressure sores, and chronic leg ulcers. Traumatic defects of the lower limb represented the largest group, with just over 100 cases. There were no specific exclusion criteria with smokers, persons with diabetes, and patients with cardiac as well as peripheral arterial and venous diseases included in the group. More than two-thirds of the cases involved a 180° rotation of the flap. There were 3 complete flap failures requiring another flap, and one further flap was converted to a free flap. Therefore, the propeller flap based on a single perforator compares well

with the success of free flaps (95%–98%) and seems to be safe provided meticulous design and technique are used.

DISCUSSION

Traditional teachings on raising pedicled or free flaps encourage us to keep a protective cuff of perivascular tissue and to avoid twisting the vascular pedicle because unprotected vessels, if twisted, are more liable to kink and lead to flap failure. Hyakusoku and colleagues[14] described an island propeller flap based on a broad central subcutaneous pedicle that can be rotated up to a maximum of 90° to release scar contractures around the flexure creases of joints. There was no attempt to locate or isolate any vascular pedicle that was assumed to be present and protected from damage within the subcutaneous pedicle. However, the restraint imposed by the thick pedicle on the extent that the flap could be rotated tended to limit its application. It would be hard to justify calling this flap a true perforator-based flap.

The propeller flap, as described here, is remarkable in that it has consistently shown that a single vascular pedicle is able to tolerate up to 180° rotation and not suffer severe vascular embarrassment each and every time. I believe the key is the way that the vascular pedicle is prepared: a radical skeletonization that divides all the fine fascial strands surrounding the vessels, in particular the venae comitantes, thereby allowing the flap to rotate comfortably up to 180°. In fact, experimental studies in rats have shown that it is possible to twist a vascular pedicle up to 360° and still maintain a viable flap.[15,16] Of course, clinically it is not necessary to rotate any flap more than 180° because one can simply twist it in the opposite direction. This twisting of the flap makes it extremely versatile when used for reconstructing local defects in many areas of the body. The indication for its use has also been extended from traumatic defects to many other conditions such as postoncologic defects, pilonidal sinuses, and pressure sores.

Over the years I have found that increasing the size of the propeller flap has allowed larger defects to be filled without any increase in the complication rate. To date, the largest defect measured 14 × 10 cm(140 cm²) and this was resurfaced with a 21 ×10 cm (210 cm²) propeller flap perfused through a single perforator artery of about 1 mm in diameter (see **Fig. 7**). The questions that remain unanswered include the correlation between size of perforator, blood flow through it, and the largest volume of tissue that it can safely sustain.

Even more intriguing than flap size is the length to width ratio of the propeller flap that can be perfused through a single perforator. Earlier, surgeons concluded that a 3:1 ratio is probably the limit of perfusion of fasciocutaneous flaps.[2,17] Donski and Fogdestam[6] postulated that the suprafascial interconnections between perforators lying along a septum effectively form an axial type flap, allowing longer flaps than otherwise to be raised. The cadaveric dissection and injection studies by Taylor and colleagues[18,19] led them to postulate that any flap based on a single vascular perforator can, in addition to sustaining its own composite block of tissue (angiosome), safely supply the angiosome of the adjacent perforator and up to half the territory of the perforator next to it. Beyond that limit, perfusion is deemed to be unreliable and necrosis is likely, especially if the delay technique has not been used. One of the longest flaps that I raised to cover a lateral calcaneal defect measured 31 × 5 cm giving it a 6:1 ratio although, being of a propeller design, the perforator was in a more central location. What I have observed in many clinical cases is that a 1-mm perforator can safely perfuse its own angiosome as well as the tissues of more than 2 vascular territories away, which is well beyond the limit of one and a half

angiosomes proposed by Taylor and colleagues. It seems logical to conclude that size of the perforator, its perfusion pressure, and the intraflap axiality of vessel arrangements are the key determinants of the length of flap that can be sustained through a particular perforator.

SUMMARY

The ability to base a flap on any perforator found in the vicinity of a wound to be reconstructed gives the surgeon unparalleled freedom when designing local flaps. The unique design of the propeller flap, pivoted around a single cleanly dissected perforator, allows the importation of truly undamaged tissue into a defect for easy closure without tension. In the lower limb this is a luxury afforded to few, if any, locally based flaps. The propeller flap is a truly versatile flap that is safe, reliable, quick to perform, and gives an agreeable aesthetic result.

ACKNOWLEDGMENTS

I acknowledge the invaluable help given to me by Bahar Gharb, MD and Antonio Rampazzo, MD in the preparation of this article.

REFERENCES

1. Ponten B. The fasciocutaneous flap: its use in soft tissue defects of the lower leg. Br J Plast Surg 1981;34(2):215–20.
2. Barclay TL, Cardoso E, Sharpe DT, et al. Repair of lower leg injuries with fascio-cutaneous flaps. Br J Plast Surg 1982;35(2):127–32.
3. Haertsch PA. The blood supply to the skin of the leg: a post-mortem investigation. Br J Plast Surg 1981; 34(4):470–7.
4. Carriquiry C, Aparecida Costa M, Vasconez LO. An anatomic study of the septocutaneous vessels of the leg. Plast Reconstr Surg 1985;76(3):354–63.
5. Gumener R, Montandon D, Marty F, et al. The subcutaneous tissue flap and the misconception on fasciocutaneous flaps. Scand J Plast Reconstr Surg 1986; 20(1):61–5.
6. Donski PK, Fogdestam I. Distally based fasciocutaneous flap from the sural region. A preliminary report. Scand J Plast Reconstr Surg 1983;17(3):191–6.
7. Amarante J, Costa H, Reis J, et al. A new distally based fasciocutaneous flap of the leg. Br J Plast Surg 1986;39(3):338–40.
8. El-Saadi MM, Khashaba AA. Three anteromedial fasciocutaneous leg island flaps for covering defects of the lower two-thirds of the leg. Br J Plast Surg 1990;43(5):536–40.
9. Shalaby HA, Higazi M, Mandour S, et al. Distally based medial island septocutaneous flap for repair

of soft-tissue defects of the lower leg. Br J Plast Surg 1991;44(3):175–8.

10. Erdmann MW, Court-Brown CM, Quaba AA. A five year review of islanded distally based fasciocutaneous flaps on the lower limb. Br J Plast Surg 1997; 50(6):421–7.

11. Teo TC. Reconstruccion de la extremidad inferior con colgaios de perforantes locales [Perforator local flaps in lower limb reconstruction]. Cir Plas Iberolatinoam 2006;32(4):287–92.

12. Inoue Y, Taylor GI. The angiosomes of the forearm: anatomic study and clinical implications. Plast Reconstr Surg 1996;98(2):195–210.

13. Matei I, Georgescu A, Chiroiu B, et al. Harvesting of forearm perforator flaps based on intraoperative vascular exploration: clinical experiences and literature review. Microsurgery 2008;28(5):321–30.

14. Hyakusoku H, Yamamoto T, Fumiiri M. The propeller flap method. Br J Plast Surg 1991;44(1):53–4.

15. Gokrem S, Sarifakioglu N, Toksoy K, et al. Effects of 360-degree pedicle torsion on island skin flaps: experimental study in rats. J Reconstr Microsurg 2005;21(5):313–6.

16. Demirseren ME, Yenidunya MO, Yenidunya S. Island rat groin flaps with twisted pedicles. Plast Reconstr Surg 2004;114(5):1190–4.

17. Tolhurst DE, Haeseker B, Zeeman RJ. The development of the fasciocutaneous flap and its clinical applications. Plast Reconstr Surg 1983; 71(5):597–606.

18. Callegari PR, Taylor GI, Caddy CM, et al. An anatomic review of the delay phenomenon: I. Experimental studies. Plast Reconstr Surg 1992;89(3): 397–407 [discussion: 417–8].

19. Taylor GI, Corlett RJ, Caddy CM, et al. An anatomic review of the delay phenomenon: II. Clinical applications. Plast Reconstr Surg 1992;89(3):408–16 [discussion: 417–8].

Pedicled Perforator Flaps in the Head and Neck

Stefan O.P. Hofer, MD, PhD, FRCS(C)[a,b,]*,
Marc A.M. Mureau, MD, PhD[c]

KEYWORDS

- Perforator flap • Head and neck reconstruction
- Superficial temporal artery perforator
- Occipital artery perforator
- Supraclavicular artery perforator
- Internal mammary artery perforator
- Facial artery perforator

Perforator flaps, since their first description in 1989,[1] have in many ways revolutionized reconstructive surgery. Whereas little more than a decade ago many surgeons were still hesitant to fully trust perforator flaps to be a reliable option, nowadays these flaps are often first choice. This early disbelief in the true value and sustainability of perforator flaps in general was nicely worded in the following section from the excellent flap book by Cormack and Lamberty[2] in 1994: "… the deep inferior epigastric artery may be dissected free of rectus abdominis while preserving 1 or 2 perforators to an island of tissue consisting only of periumbilical skin, fat, and a patch of anterior rectus sheath. Nomenclature for this variant of the musculocutaneous flap has not been universally recognized but examples are extremely few and are probably to be regarded as more a demonstration of technical skill than a significant advance in flap construction …."

The concept of perforator flaps has evolved over the years. The basic concept is that any larger named vessel in the body will give off smaller branches toward the skin on which flaps can be designed and raised as pedicled or free flaps. In the early period most, if not all, the attention regarding perforator flaps was focused on proving it was technically possible to actually dissect a very small blood vessel that perforated through a muscle and was able to vascularize a previously musculo-adipocutaneous flap as merely an adipocutaneous flap. Once this initial technical achievement had been mastered by a larger number of surgeons around the globe, further structure was brought into the new entity of perforator flap surgery. In essence there were 2 important steps to further popularize perforator flap surgery: on the one hand the further clarification of the clinical benefits and on the other hand developing classification systems to improve communication between surgeons.[3,4]

The main clinical benefits that arose from perforator flaps are twofold. In the case of a musculocutaneous perforator there is a clear donor site benefit if the innervated muscle can be left in situ. The best examples for this benefit are preservation of rectus abdominis muscle in the deep inferior epigastric perforator flap and gluteus maximus muscle in the gluteal artery perforator flaps. The second benefit was the realization that potential flaps were now all over the body and all one

[a] Division of Plastic Surgery, Department of Surgery, University Health Network, 200 Elizabeth Street, 8N-865, Toronto, ON, Canada M5G 2C4
[b] Department of Surgical Oncology, University Health Network, 200 Elizabeth Street, 8N-865, Toronto, ON, Canada M5G 2C4
[c] Oncological Reconstructive Surgery, Department of Plastic & Reconstructive Surgery, Erasmus Medical Center Rotterdam, PO Box 2040, 3000 CA Rotterdam, The Netherlands
* Corresponding author. Division of Plastic Surgery, Department of Surgery, University Health Network, 200 Elizabeth Street, 8N-865, Toronto, ON, Canada M5G 2C4.
E-mail address: stefan.hofer@uhn.on.ca

Clin Plastic Surg 37 (2010) 627–640
doi:10.1016/j.cps.2010.06.005

had to do was to find a blood vessel to raise a flap. This concept was coined "the free style perforator flap."[5] With current knowledge the concept of "free style" probably is less spectacular, because all flaps can be found and named according to their source vessels.

Once a critical mass of reconstructive surgeons had adopted perforator flaps, the lack of uniformity in classification of these new flaps became obvious. Several suggestions for classification schedules were proposed to facilitate and clarify communication between surgeons.[3,4] Classification schedules focused around 2 thoughts, on the one hand the origin of the perforator and on the other hand the course of the perforator. At present, most communications use the source vessel to describe the flap and mention whether the course of a perforator is direct, that is, from the source vessel into the skin, or indirect, that is, from the source vessel through mostly muscle into the skin.

SOURCE VESSELS FOR PERFORATOR FLAPS IN THE HEAD AND NECK

Two major arteries are responsible for the blood supply to the head and neck area. These vessels are the common carotid, which divides into external and internal carotids, and the subclavian artery. A great number of branches stem from these vessels. Many of these branches give off their own branches or perforators that in part supply the skin of the head and neck area. Not all of these branches or perforators have clinical value as source vessels for pedicled perforator flaps. Knowledge of the location of all these vessels, however, will be of great value for safe planning and execution of tissue advancements, transpositions, and rotations in the head and neck area. Those perforator branches that have clinical potential for pedicled perforator flaps are discussed here in more detail.

The first branch from the external carotid artery is the superior thyroid artery. The only vessel from the superior thyroid artery that provides blood supply to the anterior triangle of the neck skin is the sternomastoid branch. This branch can sometimes arise directly from the external carotid artery. The next is the lingual artery, which does not give off branches to the skin. The facial artery arises immediately above the lingual artery. Over its long course from its origin in the neck until its end point near the nasal root it has several branches: submental artery, premasseteric branch, inferior labial artery, superior labial artery, lateral nasal branch, and angular branch. The occipital artery arises from the posterior surface

of the external carotid artery at the level of the facial artery branch. The occipital artery gives off several perforators through the overlying muscle that supplies the skin. These perforators supply the skin in the posterior neck. The posterior auricular artery in general arises from the posterior aspect of the external carotid artery, but sometimes offshoots together with the occipital or superficial temporal artery. The auricular division of the posterior auricular artery supplies the posterior surface of the ear and the occipital division supplies the scalp posterior to the ear. The superficial temporal artery has 2 main branches, the frontal and the parietal branch. This artery has 3 main branches supplying the skin: the transverse facial artery (that sometimes arises directly from the external carotid artery), the auricular branches, and the zygomatico-orbital branches. The maxillary artery supplies skin through the infraorbital and mental branches.

The internal carotid artery supplies the skin of the face through the cutaneous branches of the ophthalmic artery, which supply the forehead through the supraorbital and supratrochlear arteries, the periorbital skin through the medial palpebral and supraorbital arteries, and part of the nasal skin through the external nasal artery. All these branches of the internal carotid artery anastomose significantly with its local counterparts from the external carotid artery.

The thyrocervical trunk of the subclavian artery gives rise to the transverse cervical artery, which has a deep and superficial branch, and the suprascapular artery. The supraclavicular artery can arise from either of these two vessels. The anatomy in this region has several exceptions with regard to the exact origin of the vessels. These vessels supply most of the skin of the neck between the clavicle and mandibular margin.

CONSIDERATIONS IN FLAP DESIGN

The goal of reconstruction with a perforator-based pedicled flap is to achieve adequate functional and aesthetic reconstruction while minimizing donor site morbidity. In the head and neck area, aesthetics play an important role for future social interaction of the patient. Detailed knowledge of the vascular possibilities in the head and neck will facilitate finding reconstructive solutions. It is important to realize that all skin transpositions, rotations, and advancements are based on perforators remaining in the raised flaps. The difference between these more traditional skin flaps and a pedicled perforator-based flap is that the latter is planned on a single perforator.

The specific use of a pedicled perforator flap in the head and neck area will depend on several considerations regarding its feasibility and usefulness. One must realize what the goal of a perforator flap is in the first place, which is to provide a flap that only contains the tissue that is really needed without harvest of any tissues that give donor site morbidity. With standard paramedian forehead flap harvest, part of the frontalis muscle is taken. A purely adipocutaneous paramedian forehead flap could be coined a perforator flap. The fact is that harvest of part of the frontalis muscle does not give significant donor site morbidity but it does aid in the safer circulation of the flap. Therefore, even though a perforator flap could be raised in this location it adds only risk and no benefit. In addition, simply closing a defect with a pedicled perforator flap because it is technically feasible does not necessarily fit the philosophy of aesthetic facial reconstruction. For example, in the case of a facial artery perforator (FAP) flap, the thicker skin from the nasolabial fold makes an unfavorable match for the very thin skin of the periorbital region.

The limitations of primary closure after flap harvest in the head and neck area limit the size and locations for pedicled perforator flaps. Donor site closure with a skin graft, as can be performed on the extremities, should generally not be done in most of the anterior face and neck. The best areas for pedicled perforator flap harvest to the head and neck area are the upper trunk, neck, and nasolabial regions where vessels pass through and some skin laxity is available. However, the temporoparietal area has slightly less laxity and can supply adequate skin for an islanded flap, and the question is whether the vessels in this location should be called perforators because they are cutaneous vessels. The occipital area does have true muscular perforators, which can be incorporated into a perforator flap design; however, the limitations in skin laxity and possible flap movement make primary closure with meaningful flap movement difficult.

Two flap designs are conceivable for perforator flaps in the head and neck area. First, the islanded flap can be moved over a smaller distance depending on the length of its perforator or over a longer distance if the source vessel is cut and used in lengthening the pedicle. Cutting of the source vessel in the head and neck area is an acceptable technique because the area is extremely rich in vascularization and is not limited to 2 or 3 major blood vessels such as in the upper or lower extremity. Second, an islanded flap can be moved as a propeller-type flap.

CLINICAL APPLICATIONS OF PERFORATOR-BASED PEDICLED FLAPS IN THE HEAD AND NECK AREA

The design and execution of perforator-based pedicled flaps in the head and neck area is truly an example of free-style perforator flap surgery, with countless possibilities in theory. Some possibilities are more useful than others, and the following sections present a few of the more applicable options in more detail.

FACIAL ARTERY–BASED PERFORATOR FLAPS
Submental Artery Perforator Flap
Background
Martin and colleagues[6] first described the submental flap in 1993. In their quest for an ideal flap to restore facial defects with regard to color, contour, and tissue texture they identified the submental artery as a consistent pedicle of adequate length for an anterior neck skin flap. The submental flap has an inconspicuous donor site if designed correctly and can be used as a cutaneous, myocutaneous, fasciocutaneous, or osteofasciocutaneous flap for facial and intraoral defects.

Anatomy
The submental artery is a consistent branch that arises below the lower mandibular border deep to the submandibular gland in the neck. This vessel, with a 1.0- to 2.0-mm diameter at its origin, runs forward over the mylohyoid muscle turning around the mandibular border to end on the surface of the chin where it anastomoses with the mental artery and inferior labial arteries. The submental artery gives off 1 to 4 small perforators that supply the platysma muscle and the skin over the submental triangle. The vessels of one side anastomose with the contralateral side, thus providing blood supply to the submental skin. For a useful arc of rotation the source vessel rather than only the perforators needs to be used and, although the platysma muscle is classically incorporated into the flap for safer circulation, it can be raised as a true perforator flap, sparing the platsyma muscle.[7] The anterior belly of the digastric muscle has been reported to lie superior of the vessel in 70% of cases and is usually incorporated in the flap. The venous drainage of the submental flap is from the submental vein into the facial vein and then into the common facial vein. From here it can drain into the external and internal jugular vein.

Planning and surgical dissection
The flap is designed at least 1 cm below the mandibular margin to avoid any visible scarring

on the face when closing the donor site defect. The flap design is always elliptical to allow simple primary closure. With the patient looking forward and the neck in a neutral position, a pinch test is performed to assess the amount of laxity of the anterior neck skin and decide on the flap width that will allow primary closure. The flap length runs between the mandibular angles. Flap sizes as large as 18 × 8 cm have been reported.[8]

Flap harvest has been reported in several different manners. The approach can be from ipsilateral or contralateral and from superior or inferior. One preferred method is to make an ipsilateral inferior incision through skin and platysma, and dissect the submandibular gland carefully off the prospective flap. The submental and facial arteries are identified. Then the inferior incision is carried on and around the contralateral superior side. The flap is now raised in the subplatysmal plane from contralateral. Superiorly care must be taken to stay tight to the platysma muscle to prevent marginal mandibular nerve branch damage. Once on the ipsilateral side, dissection will include the anterior belly of the digastric muscle, as the pedicle runs deep to this muscle in 70% of cases. In case the flap needs to be tunneled to the oral cavity, the underlying mylohyoid muscle will have to be cut partially or entirely. Care needs to be taken not to dissect the skin flap of the pedicle, as the pedicle runs very deep. While keeping the flap under tension the pedicle is dissected to its origin.

Pedicle dissection should only be performed until tension-free inset is possible. In the case of more pedicle length being required, several scenarios are possible. The facial vessels distal to the submental branch can be cut, the facial vein can be cut and anastomosed at the recipient site, additional length of the vein can be achieved by cutting the common facial vein and letting outflow pass through anastomoses through the external jugular vein, and finally the facial vessels can be cut proximally thus creating a retrograde flow submental flap. A retrograde perfused submental flap should preferably be inset without any tension whatsoever to prevent further venous compromise.

Special considerations
The submental flap can be harvested as a free flap, which prevents any arc of rotation problems. However, as a pedicled flap it is versatile, supplying tissue of good quality for facial reconstruction. One area of interest is the use of the submental flap for intraoral reconstruction after ablative cancer resection. There remains some difference in opinion regarding the suitability of the submental flap in the presence of node-positive disease. The opponents of its use believe that saving the submental vessels compromises level 1 node dissection. Level 1 nodes consist of the submental and submandibular nodes, which often are involved in oral cancer. Proponents indicate that careful dissection and saving of the vascular pedicle of the submental flap before or during node dissection does not negatively influence local control or survival.

FAP Flap

Background
Nasolabial flaps are based on the facial artery, and can be superiorly or inferiorly pedicled. The flaps have been used as skin flaps or as musculomucosal flaps for either skin or intraoral lining defects. The pedicle can be subcutaneous, as an islanded flap, to prevent a second stage for pedicle division. The FAP flap, which is supplied by the perforating branches of the facial artery, has been a further refinement of the use of the nasolabial skin.[9] This flap was the first true perforator flap described that could be raised in the face.

Originally the FAP flap was described for reconstruction of perioral defects. The flap can reach the lateral cheek or lower eyelid. However, this would not be a first choice for reconstruction of these areas because it does not provide optimal tissue and causes scars, keeping in mind the unit principles of aesthetic facial reconstruction. The perioral region, on the other hand, is ideal for the FAP flap, as it enables reconstruction of an upper lip unit with minimal donor site morbidity. The FAP flap is harvested from the jowl area, which especially in the older patient has adequate skin stock. The jowl is an area of considerable skin laxity, which in a different patient population also is corrected when facial rejuvenation surgery is requested.

Due to rich collateral circulation in the face, these flaps have been used successfully following neck dissection in patients with atherosclerotic disease, and following pre- and postablative irradiation. Problems with tip necrosis in these flaps have been experienced in patients who did not stop smoking. The only absolute contraindication is insufficient skin laxity, either because the defect is too large or because a similar local flap has been used before.

Anatomy
The domain of the FAP flap runs between the points where the facial artery curves around the mandible to the alar base, even though the facial artery continues on to the medial canthus. In the area from the lower border of the mandible to the angle of the mouth, the facial artery is easy to dissect in comparison with the area above the corner of the mouth where it runs through the facial

muscles. Apart from the few named branches coming off the facial artery as described previously, a great number of unnamed branches or perforators arise from the facial artery. In the area between the lower border of the mandible and the alar base, the facial artery on average gives off approximately 6 perforators with an average vessel diameter of 1.2 mm and an average length of 2.5 cm. The flap does not interfere with facial nerve function, as it is harvested where no major facial nerve branches run.

Planning and surgical dissection

Handheld Doppler investigation should be performed to identify the exact course of the facial artery (**Figs. 1–3**). The perforators that come off the facial artery supplying the facial skin cannot often be reliably identified because of the high background volume of the source vessel. A slight crescendo indicating a FAP can sometimes be heard; however, this is uncommon. Application of computed tomographic angiography has not been used for this specific application, yet may give helpful information for surgical planning in selected cases. After the precise course of the facial artery is known a flap design can be made.

Defect assessment and, if required, preparation for reconstruction by adapting the defect to the unit principles of aesthetic facial reconstruction is performed. A foil template is then used to mark part or the entire unit to be reconstructed. This template is then marked as the prospective flap on the skin of the jowl area over the course of the facial artery. Identifying a FAP through either an exploratory incision along one side of the planned flap or subcutaneous careful blunt vertically-oriented dissection from the wound edge of the adjacent defect checks the final feasibility of the planned flap. The plane of dissection is above the facial musculature, which should be visible in the more cranial part of the dissection. Once a FAP is identified, its suitability for the projected flap is assessed by evaluating the possible arc of rotation that the flap would have with this perforator. If the arc of rotation is deemed inadequate, one should look for another perforator or change the flap design. In the unlikely case that no suitable perforator can be identified, a conversion to a classic nasolabial flap is an option; however, these flaps also obtain their blood supply from multiple perforating vessels from the facial artery.

Once a specific FAP has been selected, the flap can be cut and raised in a plane above the facial muscles. Dissection of the pedicle is performed only so far that a good transposition into the defect is enabled without leaving unnecessary bulk at the pedicle requiring secondary thinning. Rarely does a clearly identifiable vein run with the FAP. The reason for this is that the facial vein runs well posterior to the facial artery together with the pre-masseteric branch arising from the facial artery. Most of the time venous drainage will be from the fibrofatty tissue around the artery, similar to the situation in digital neurovascular island flaps. A clearly identifiable artery with a small amount of fatty tissue around it should form the pedicle of the flap. The flap can be rotated up to 180° while retaining adequate vascularity.

Finally, the flap is positioned into the defect with little tension. At the end of the operation, the flap often has the classic blue shimmer of slight to moderate venous congestion, and will swell slightly in the postoperative phase. Inset with minimal tension is therefore beneficial for postoperative

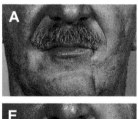
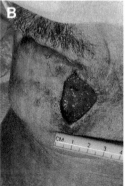
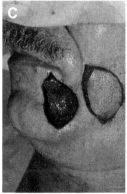
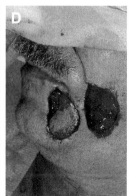
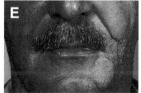

Fig. 1. (*A*) Appearance after primary closure of large basal cell skin cancer in the left mental area. The patient had problems eating and was drooling because of the excessively tight closure. (*B*) Recreation of the defect by releasing scar tissue allowing eversion of the left lower lip. (*C*) Execution of a FAP flap in the left jowl area to recruit the excessive lax skin for the defect. (*D*) Inset FAP flap. (*E*) One year follow-up result showing adequate lower lip positioning, giving subsequent relief of symptoms.

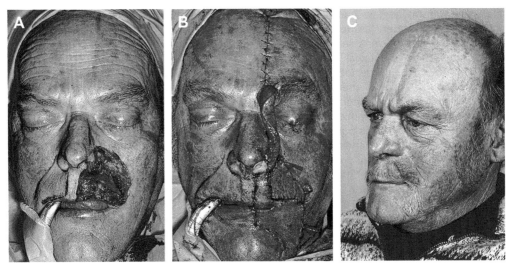

Fig. 2. (*A*) Large squamous cell cancer defect of left upper lip region. (*B*) Reconstruction of individual aesthetic units with a FAP flap for the upper lip region, a paramedian forehead flap for the nasal defect, and an extended lip-switch flap for the upper lip vermillion and nasal floor deficit. (*C*) three-year follow-up result.

circulation. The donor site is closed primarily after local undermining of the cheek.

Special considerations

The unit principles of aesthetic facial reconstruction in combination with flap dissection with a good circulation will achieve good results. A well-circulated flap can be obtained by taking into account the size of the flap in relation to the

size and location of entry into the flap of the perforator. Perforators with a diameter similar to those of the facial artery have been reported to supply areas of skin measuring 5 × 10 cm.[10,11] The FAP flap generally requires maximum transposition to reach the defect. Most of the time, therefore, the perforator vessel will enter the flap at one edge of the flap, as in a propeller flap. The perforator can in theory support a flap size of 5 × 5 cm. For

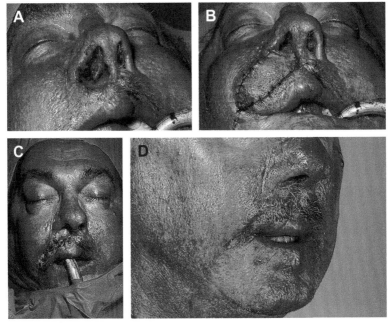

Fig. 3. (*A*) Nasal floor defect after basal cell cancer resection in a patient with a previous bilateral cleft lip and palate repair. The defect resulted in an oronasal fistula, which required a more bulky flap to enable closure of the fistula defect. (*B*) FAP flap rotated into the defect on one perforator. (*C*) Second-stage revision of excessive skin after closure of fistula and defect. (*D*) Early result 6 months after second-stage revision.

clinical application this size is larger than primary closure in the jowl area would allow.

Bulky flaps can be thinned; however, care should be taken to avoid aggressive thinning of the flap for the sake of a one-stage perfect result within the end of a partially necrotic flap. Pedicle thinning to bury the pedicle invisibly is sufficient if possible in stage 1.

Superficial Temporal Artery–Based Perforator Flaps

Background

Flaps on the superficial temporal artery have been well investigated and used over the past century. Countless variations of forehead and scalping flaps based on this vessel have been devised. It can be debated whether the superficial temporal artery is a perforator, because it does pierce the deep fascia; however, the superficial temporal artery really is a continuation of the same vessel. On the other hand it may also be classified as a direct perforator that travels into the skin. Unlike some of the other perforator flaps, this flap bears little novelty as it has been well documented. Its main use in current practice is the large surface area that can be obtained for covering exposed bone by using the fascia without the skin, which allows for primary donor site closure. The fascia can then be skin grafted. The other less frequent use is as a smaller hair-bearing flap for eyebrow or mustache reconstruction whereby the donor site can also be closed primarily. Large scalp flaps are less commonly used in practice because microsurgical possibilities have largely replaced these flaps.

Anatomy

The superficial temporal artery is not a true perforator, as this vessel starts deep to or within the parotid gland and then in its course, as it ascends behind the ascending ramus of the mandible, pierces the deep fascia 4 to 5 mm in front of the tragus. From there onward it has a superficial course as it divides 2 to 4 cm above the zygomatic arch into frontal (anterior) and parietal (posterior) branches. The parietal branch is most feasible to serve as pedicle for a superficial temporal artery–based flap. The parietal branch runs within a 2-cm band centered on the auditory canal. The artery continues cranially and anastomoses with its contralateral branch. The superficial temporal vein runs most often posterior to the artery. Over its course between piercing the deep fascia and dividing into the aforementioned branches, a few other named branches arise from the superficial temporal artery supplying the periorbital and auricular region. For a superficial temporal artery based

flap, skin or fascia overlying the vessels can be used.

The blood supply to the cranial aspect of the auricle and the mastoid region is derived from the posterior auricular and superficial temporal arteries. Various flaps designed to move retroauricular skin on a pedicle containing branches of the superficial temporal artery have been described.[12–14] The anatomic vascular basis of the retroauricular flap based on the superficial temporal artery depends on 2 sets of anastomoses. First, on the cranial surface of the auricle, auricular anastomoses exist between auricular branches derived from the superficial temporal artery and posterior auricular artery. Second, in the scalp superior to the ear, scalp anastomoses occur between the parietal branch and the terminal branches of the posterior auricular artery.[15]

Planning and surgical dissection

Preoperatively, the course of the parietal branch of the superficial temporal artery is marked using a handheld Doppler. In case of a hair-bearing fasciocutaneous island flap for eyebrow (**Fig. 4**) or mustache reconstruction, a template of the eyebrow or upper lip defect is made. This exact template of the defect is used to plan the skin island directly above the parietal branch. Next, the skin is incised 1 to 2 cm posterior to the parietal branch of the superficial temporal artery to limit the risk of damaging the vessel. The skin of the scalp is raised just below the hair follicles and the flap is elevated with 0.5 to 1.5 cm superficial temporoparietal fascial tissue preserved around the artery and concomitant vein.[16] The skin island is incised, including the underlying temporoparietal fascia, after which the flap can be raised on its pedicle, which can be dissected up to the root of the helix.[17] The flap can be transferred to the defect through a subcutaneous tunnel, which must be wide enough to prevent venous congestion.

In the case of periorbital defect reconstructions, a fasciocutaneous island flap based on the frontal branch of the superficial temporal artery is also possible. Care must be taken, however, not to damage the temporal branch of the facial nerve.[17] Clear disadvantages of this flap are the conspicuous donor site scar on the forehead and asymmetry of brow position as a result of primary donor site closure, which does not make it the flap of first choice for these types of defects.

For reconstruction of forehead or periorbital defects with exposed bone the superficial temporal artery, a perforator flap can also be used as a fascial flap, which is subsequently covered with a full-thickness skin graft (**Fig. 5**).

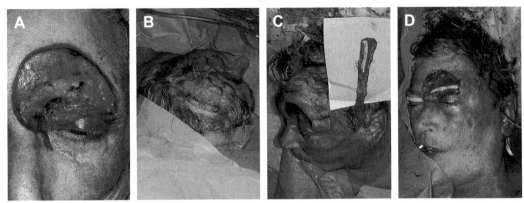

Fig. 4. (*A*) Periorbital defect with exposed frontal bone after wide local excision of a Merkel cell carcinoma. (*B*) The fasciocutaneous superficial temporal artery flap is marked using an exact template for brow reconstruction. (*C*) The flap on its pedicle containing the superficial temporal vessels. A strip of 2 cm fascia around the vessels was included, and the size of the fascial part containing the cutaneous island equaled the periorbital defect to cover the frontal bone. (*D*) Immediate postoperative result after inset of the flap through a wide subcutaneous tunnel. The upper lid defect was closed with a full-thickness skin graft of the contralateral upper lid. The frontal defect was covered with a supraclavicular full-thickness skin graft.

After Doppler identification of the course of the parietal branch, the skin is incised 1 to 2 cm posterior to the artery and elevated just below the hair follicles. A Y incision is made over the temporoparietal fascia to minimize undermining. After dissection of the total temporoparietal fascia, a flap length of 12 to 14 cm and a flap width of 6 to 10 cm can be achieved.[16] The pedicle of the flap is dissected up to the helical root and the flap is transposed to the defect through a subcutaneous tunnel.

In the case of a retroauricular flap, which can be used for reconstruction of defects of the nose, ears, socket, eyelids, eyebrows, malar region, and forehead, the superficial artery and its branches are marked first using a handheld Doppler. This flap can either be raised anterograde on the superficial temporal artery,[12] as a reversed flow flap on the parietal branch of the superficial artery,[18] or on the superior auricular artery, which also branches off the superficial temporal artery just above the root of the ear.[13] An elliptical skin

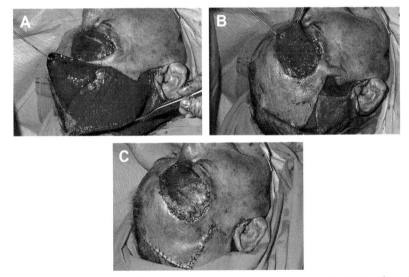

Fig. 5. (*A*) Large-defect right forehead with exposed bone after basal cell cancer resection. The temporoparietal fascia is dissected free with the temporoparietal vessels as a guide. (*B*) Temporoparietal artery–based fascia flap to cover large defect. No skin is taken, as the size of the defect would otherwise not allow primary donor site closure and bring hair to the forehead. (*C*) Split-thickness skin grafting of the temporoparietal fascial surface.

island including the posterior auricular and mastoid region is planned, with the retroauricular sulcus marking the midline of the flap. A hairy scalp strip may also be included if needed. Next, a T incision is made in the temporal region and the skin overlying the superficial temporal fascia is elevated in a subfollicular plane. A transverse incision is made above the helical root, and a subfollicular dissection of the scalp is continued anteriorly with a facelift dissection plane in front of the ear. To protect the superior auricular artery and concomitant veins, meticulous dissection of the skin island is performed in a subaponeurotic plane just above the perichondrium.[18] In addition, perivascular tissue of 2.5 to 3 cm around the superior auricular artery is left intact as a subcutaneous pedicle. In the case of a reversed flow flap, dissection proceeds until the zygomatic arch is reached, below which the superficial temporal vessels are ligated and cut (below where the superior auricular artery arises). The frontal branch is also ligated and cut proximally, after which the parietal branch with 3 cm perivascular fascial tissue is elevated in a subfascial plane and used as a pedicle. The pivot point is then located on or just below the temporal crest.[18] Finally, a wide subcutaneous tunnel is made along a straight line between the pedicle base and the defect through which the flap is passed without tension. The donor site defect can be minimized by a face-lift type incision and undermining of the neck, after which the defect is covered with a skin graft.[13]

Special considerations

Although dissection of the superficial temporal artery perforator flap is generally straightforward, a potential pitfall is the absence of the superficial temporal vein. Occasionally the vein lies up to 3 cm posterior to the superficial temporal artery. Therefore, if the vein is not found centrally in the pedicle, it may be located more posteriorly, very close to the tragus and upper pole of the ear.[16]

If the dissection of the skin is performed too superficially, hair follicles may be damaged, causing alopecia. This complication occurs most commonly in an area approximately 0.5 to 1 cm in front of and behind the incision line, and may require scar revision in a later procedure.[16]

The size of the skin islands of the fasciocutaneous flap design is limited to make primary closure of the donor site still possible. A flap width up to 3 cm usually allows for primary closure of the donor site. Temporary venous congestion of these fasciocutaneous island flaps is regularly encountered, but usually resolves after 4 to 7 days.[17]

The most important complication related to the retroauricular island flaps is venous congestion, which requires leeching or bleeding.[18] It has been suggested that venous congestion by either an inevitable torsion in the pedicle[19] or unfavorable physiology[19,20] is the main cause. Another disadvantage of these flaps is the limited amount of skin available; therefore they are only suitable for small to medium-sized facial defects.[18]

Occipital Artery–Based Perforator Flaps

Background

Occipital artery–based perforator flaps have been reported for improvement of scar contracture or salvage surgery after major skin breakdown and bony exposure in the neck. Especially in male patients, the hair-bearing quality of these flaps enables restoration of a beard. The tightness of the scalp makes any flap with a larger width impossible to close, making skin grafting for the donor site defect necessary.

Anatomy

The occipital artery arises opposite to the facial artery on the posterior surface of the external carotid artery. It runs posterior across the internal jugular vein and deep to the posterior belly of the digastric muscle, continuing in a submuscular course until it pierces the fascia between the sternomastoid and trapezius muscles. As it pierces the fascia it provides 3 perforator branches that supply the skin. These branches have a descending, transverse, and ascending course, and can be used individually to serve as pedicle for an occipital artery–based perforator flap.

Planning and surgical dissection

Handheld Doppler investigation should be performed to assess the exact course of the occipital artery. When a large flap with an intact skin base is taken, the Doppler will confirm patency of the occipital artery. If a smaller flap is used, the exact location of the occipital artery perforator will aid in precise planning for an islanded flap. These flaps can potentially reach the anterior chin; however, as islanded perforator flaps the more likely indications would be posterior scalp defects of limited size with bony exposure or defects, for example after infection, local burn, or pressure sore. In those cases the excess skin that is available in the neck, allowing primary closure, would be amenable to a propeller-type rotation to cover exposed bone.

After identification of an adequate Doppler signal in a location that will allow flap rotation into the defect, an exploratory incision along one edge of the flap or careful dissection from the wound edge can be performed to identify an adequate perforator on which to base the flap.

Once a perforator is identified, the flap is cut and raised in the subfascial or supragaleal plane. After full dissection the flap is rotated into the defect up to 180°. Flap inset has to be with limited tension to the rotated vascular pedicle. The vascular pedicle should be released as far as easy rotation will allow.

Special considerations

The advantage that this flap has for a man who wants hair restored in the neck is a disadvantage when used for a woman, and makes it less suitable. These flaps, when large, should be reserved for very selected and salvage cases, because more elegant solutions with anterior local or free tissue transfers are available.

Supraclavicular Artery–Based Perforator Flaps

Background

In situations for which healthy local tissue for reconstruction of facial or neck defects is not available (eg, after burns or radiation), other donor sites can be considered. The shoulder area is potentially a suitable distant donor site from where a thin fasciocutaneous flap with an acceptable match in skin color and texture, especially for the lower face, neck, and upper chest wall region, can be elevated. In 1842, Mutter first described a random pattern flap of the supraclavicular region that extended toward the shoulder.[21] After closer examination of the vascularization, the flap was described as a supraclavicular axial pattern flap.[22] Anatomically, this neck/shoulder flap was based on the supraclavicular artery. Recently, renewed attention was focused on the supraclavicular flap with a study of its surgical anatomy, surgical technique, and clinical application for postburn facial and neck defect reconstructions.[23] Its application for postoncologic head and neck reconstruction, including tracheostoma and hypopharynx defect reconstructions, has been reported.[24,25] In addition to the pedicled supraclavicular artery island flap, a true perforator-free supraclavicular flap has recently been described for head and neck reconstructions.[26,27]

Anatomy

The supraclavicular artery arises 3 to 4 cm from the origin of the transverse cervical artery beneath or lateral to the posterior part of the omohyoid muscle.[28] The artery can always be found in the triangle between the dorsal edge of the sternocleidomastoid muscle, the external jugular vein, and the medial part of the clavicle. Usually the artery branches off about 3 cm above the clavicle at a distance of 8 to 10 cm from the sternoclavicular joint, approximately 2 to 3 cm dorsal to the sternocleidomastoid muscle. The mean diameter of the artery is about 1.5 mm. The artery is always accompanied by a concomitant vein, which drains into the transverse cervical vein, and has a diameter of about 2 to 3 mm. Very often there is also a second vein, which is a branch of the external jugular vein with a diameter of about 2.5 mm. The vascular territory of the supraclavicular artery extends from the supraclavicular region to the ventral surface of the deltoid muscle. The surface can vary from 10 to 16 cm in width to 22 to 30 cm in length.[28]

There are 3 to 5 perforators coursing through the platysma to the skin, which come from the superficial branch of the transverse cervical artery, the transverse cervical artery itself, or from the deep branch. These perforators are independent from the supraclavicular artery, which has a separate course parallel to the clavicle toward the shoulder. Of the transverse cervical artery and its branches, 1 or 2 concomitant veins and a superficial cervical vein are consistently present. Venous perforators accompanying the arterial ones always drain into the superficial cervical vein, which connects to the external jugular vein.[28]

Planning and surgical dissection

The supraclavicular vessels are marked using a handheld Doppler probe. Next, the pedicle and flap are outlined (**Fig. 6**). During flap elevation the patient rests on his or her side at a 45° angle. The incision is taken down to the deltoid muscle in a subfascial plane and the flap is raised from lateral to medial. In the medial third of the flap the pedicle can easily be identified by transillumination. Reaching the previously outlined medial edge of the required skin island, the skin is incised superficially, taking care not to damage the pedicle at the supraclavicular level.[23,24] Further preparation of the pedicle is superior at the subcutaneous level, forming a tunnel, and inferior of the pedicle at the subfascial level. Dissection can be continued to the pivot point at the origin of the supraclavicular artery.[23,24] The aim of preparing a tunnel is to avoid visible scars on the medial part of the neck; however, if there is too much compression of the pedicle the flap may be inset without making a tunnel[25,28] or as a classic pedicled tubed flap, making a second stage necessary.[29] After inset of the flap, the donor site can usually be closed primarily after extensive subcutaneous undermining of the wound edges, supposedly even in extreme wide flaps of up to 16 cm.[23,24] In the case of a free supraclavicular perforator flap, the lateral caudal margin of the flap is incised through the superficial cervical fascia until the omohyoid muscle is identified and retracted or cut to achieve optimal exposure of

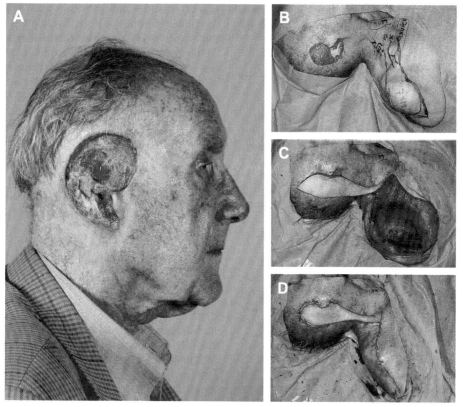

Fig. 6. (*A*) Large retroauricular defect with exposed skull bone after ear amputation and Mohs excision of a basal cell carcinoma. (*B*) Outline of a right supraclavicular artery flap measuring 6 × 19 cm. The supraclavicular artery pierces the fascia in the triangle formed by the sternocleidomastoid muscle, external jugular vein, and clavicle. (*C*) After elevation of the flap and wide undermining of the donor site wound edges. (*D*) Immediate postoperative result after the first stage. The pedicle of the flap is tubed and will be severed and inset 3 weeks later.

the transverse cervical artery, which runs beneath the muscle.[26] Laterally the superficial cervical vein is identified and followed to posterior. After the external jugular vein is identified and divided, the superficial cervical vein is cut beyond the flap's limit. At this point, dissection goes back to the transverse cervical artery, which is followed to the trapezius muscle. The deep branch of the transverse cervical artery is divided after the spinal accessory nerve is identified and preserved. The medial and deep surfaces of the vessel are dissected free, taking care not to injure the brachial plexus, which lies underneath the proximal third of the vessel, and leaving a cuff of fibrofatty tissue around the perforators. The vessels are then followed to their origin and cut. At this point, the flap potentially has 2 alternative vascular pedicles, anteromedial and posterolateral, that could also allow for flow-through applications. The length of the pedicle usually ranges between 3 and 6 cm. Pedicle caliber ranges between 1.5 and 2.5 mm for the artery and between 2 and 3 mm for the superficial cervical vein.[26]

Special considerations

To increase size (especially in children whose cheek area is large and supraclavicular area is small) the supraclavicular flap may be preexpanded first.[23,29] After a period of 3 months, when the flap has the desired size and the capsule has matured, it may be transferred as an island flap or as a peninsular flap, which needs to be divided and inset 2 weeks later.[29]

In the case of postoncologic head and neck reconstruction, harvesting a supraclavicular flap is contraindicated if an ipsilateral level 5 neck dissection has also been performed. When one side of the neck has previously been irradiated or operated on, the contralateral shoulder is used to avoid the frustration of scar tissue dissection.[25] To minimize the chance of venous congestion or partial flap necrosis, tunneling of the supraclavicular island flap under radiated tissue or areas of previous scarring is not recommended.[24,25]

Flap size of the free supraclavicular perforator flap is limited to allow for primary closure, and the pedicle may be short (3.5–5 cm). It can be used for selected cases of oral or facial reconstruction, but the flap is absolutely contraindicated in cases of ipsilateral neck metastases and in irradiated necks.[26]

Internal Mammary Artery Perforator Flap

Background
The deltopectoral and pectoralis major flaps traditionally have been the workhorse pedicled regional flaps for soft-tissue reconstruction of head and neck defects. The deltopectoral flap, however, leaves a significant donor site defect, which usually requires an unsightly skin graft, and its pedicle needs to be severed with further inset of the flap at a second stage. The pectoralis major flap can be bulky, providing poor contour, and can lead to secondary contractures of the pedicle causing restricted neck mobility.[30]

A variation of the deltopectoral flap, based on perforators of the internal mammary artery and allowing islanding of this flap, was developed by Neligan and colleagues,[31] which they consequently have called the internal mammary artery perforator (IMAP) flap.[30]

Anatomy
The internal mammary artery arises from the first part of the subclavian artery. It runs 1 to 2 cm lateral to the edge of the sternum and divides into the deep superior epigastric and the musculophrenic arteries between the sixth costal cartilage and the sixth intercostal space. It is accompanied in its distal part by 2 concomitant veins, which usually merge between the third and fourth intercostal spaces to form one internal mammary vein, which ascends to drain into the brachiocephalic vein.[30]

A cutaneous perforating branch passes through the intercostal muscles and the medial fibers of pectoralis major to supply the overlying skin in a segmental manner. This IMAP branches off the internal mammary artery in the first 5 to 6 intercostal spaces. The perforator pedicle usually consists of one artery and one vein, with an accompanying nerve, the anterior cutaneous branch of the corresponding intercostal nerve.[30]

The first to fifth IMAPs give segmental supply to the skin of the ventromedial thorax, reaching from the skin overlying the clavicle down to below the inframammary fold. There usually is an overlap of supplied skin zones between consecutive perforators. The first IMAP supplies the skin caudal to the jugulum, the sternoclavicular joint, and the medial third of the clavicle. The zone craniomedial to the areola is nourished by the second IMAP. The nipple areola complex and medial conjoining skin is most frequently supplied by the third or the second and third IMAPs. The fourth IMAP usually supplies the skin inferior to the areola

cranially to the inframammary fold. The skin of the proximal abdominal wall caudally to the inframammary fold is nourished by the fifth IMAP.[32]

In a recent anatomic study the mean size of all skin areas was about 13 × 7 cm.[32] The largest detected skin dimensions were on average 16 × 9 cm for the second IMAP, with a maximum of 20 × 13 cm. Supplied areas of IMAP 1, 3, and 4 were of comparable mean size. The smallest skin area was supplied by IMAP 5 and measured 8 × 4 cm on average.[32] The sizes of these vascular territories correspond well to the mean diameter of the IMAPs, which range from 1.1 mm for the fifth IMAP to 1.6 mm for the second IMAP.[32] The diameter of the accompanying veins ranges between 1.5 and 3.2 mm.[33]

Planning and surgical dissection
Preoperatively, the IMAPs at the second, third, and fourth intercostal spaces along the sternal border on each side are located using a handheld Doppler device (**Fig. 7**).[30,34] The side chosen depends on the location of the defect. For a centrally located defect, the side with a stronger Doppler signal is chosen. Then the flap is designed with its long axis parallel to the intercostal space. Preferably, the second IMAP is chosen unless the Doppler signal is significantly weaker than that at the third intercostal space.[34] A bilateral flap can be raised if required.[30]

The superior incision is made first, down to the fascia. Subfascial dissection proceeds inferiorly until the IMAP vessels are identified.[34] The perforator vessels are dissected and assessed for suitability and size, judged by visualizing a pulsatile artery and a vein approaching 1 mm in diameter.[30] Next, the flap is fully incised and islanded. The pectoralis major muscle attachments cranial to the perforators can be divided to increase pedicle length.[34] Removal of the costal cartilage caudal to the perforator has been reported to gain access to the distal internal mammary vessels, for ligation and division in order to maximize the reach of the flap.[30,31] The flap is then rotated to reconstruct the defect, either through a subcutaneous tunnel or by dividing the narrow skin bridge between the donor site and the defect.[31,34] The donor site is closed primarily, if needed, by means of a chevron advancement of the lower chest skin in the case of bilateral flaps.[30]

Special considerations
An IMAP flap can be based on any of the perforators, provided that the accompanying vein is of adequate size. Flaps based on the upper 4 perforators are most useful for head and neck reconstruction; however, flaps based on the fifth, sixth, or even the seventh perforators can be used for other indications, including chest wall reconstruction. After

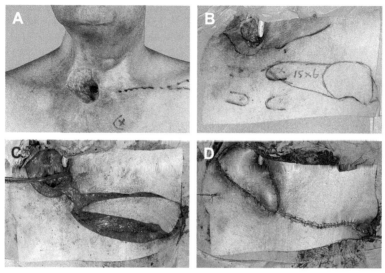

Fig. 7. (*A*) Paratracheostomal defect and osteoradionecrosis of the proximal clavicle after total laryngectomy and postoperative radiotherapy. (*B*) A left IMAP flap measuring 15 × 6 cm is planned based on the first perforator of the internal mammary artery. (*C*) Intraoperative view after radical debridement of the wound and necrotic clavicle. The IMAP flap is islanded on the first perforator. (*D*) Immediate postoperative view after rotation and inset of the IMAP flap. The donor site was closed primarily.

the fifth rib there is a conjoint costal cartilage, which becomes much more difficult to dissect and may limit the dissection of the lowermost perforator.[30]

The IMAP flap can be safely raised on one perforator as an island flap, which can be rotated up to 180°, while maintaining primary closure of the donor site. If there is any concern over the size of the perforator a second adjacent perforator should be taken. Provided the internal mammary artery is adequately mobilized after ligating and dividing it distally, no problems with twisting or kinking of the pedicle have been reported.[30,31]

Because there is considerable overlap between the vascular territories of the adjacent perforators,[32] the IMAP flap can be designed transversely, vertically, or obliquely.[30] In the neck region its long pedicle makes it suitable for pharyngeal and tracheostoma reconstruction, tracheoesophageal fistula repair, and anterior neck resurfacing.[30,31,34] The size limits of the IMAP flap are the sternal midline to just beyond the anterior axillary line. Therefore, without prior delay of an extension, the flap will not reach above the jawline reliably.[30] Similar to pectoralis major flaps, its use in women needs careful assessment because displacement of the breast may occur.[30]

SUMMARY

The continuing interest in surgical anatomy for reconstructive procedures has given a tremendous boost to the further development and refinement of reconstructive surgery of the head and neck.

Over the past 2 decades significant changes in the understanding of vascular anatomy of pedicled flaps in the head and neck area have led to the discovery and development of several very useful flaps. These flaps have contributed to improved functional and aesthetic outcomes for head and neck reconstruction while preserving donor site function. We have to remain critical, however, of their advances and realize that not every reconstruction will require or benefit from a perforator flap, as previously well-established nonperforator flaps still have their indication and can give excellent results. The most important skill in reconstructive surgery of the head and neck is not cutting the flap, but assessing the defect, planning the reconstruction, and choosing wisely from the ever-increasing options available.

REFERENCES

1. Koshima I, Soeda S. Inferior epigastric artery skin flaps without rectus abdominis muscle. Br J Plast Surg 1989;42(6):645–8.
2. Cormack GC, Lamberty BGH. The arterial anatomy of skin flaps. 2nd edition. London: Churchill, Livingstone; 1994.
3. Geddes CR, Morris SF, Neligan PC. Perforator flaps: evolution, classification, and applications. Ann Plast Surg 2003;50(1):90–9.
4. Blondeel PN, Van Landuyt KH, Monstrey SJ, et al. The "Gent" consensus on perforator flap terminology: preliminary definitions. Plast Reconstr Surg 2003; 112(5):1378–83.

5. Wei FC, Mardini S. Free style free flaps. Plast Reconstr Surg 2004;114(4):910–6.

6. Martin D, Pascal JF, Baudet J, et al. The submental island flap: a new donor site. Anatomy and clinical applications as a free or pedicled flap. Plast Reconstr Surg 1993;92(5):867–73.

7. Ishihara T, Igata T, Masuguchi S, et al. Submental perforator flap: location and number of submental perforating vessels. Scand J Plast Reconstr Surg Hand Surg 2008;42(3):127–31.

8. Pistre V, Pelissier P, Martin D, et al. Ten years of experience with the submental flap. Plast Reconstr Surg 2001;108(6):1576–81.

9. Hofer SO, Posch NA, Smit X. The facial artery perforator flap for reconstruction of perioral defects. Plast Reconstr Surg 2005;115(4):996–1003.

10. Koshima I, Nanba Y, Tsutsui T, et al. Perforator flaps in lower extremity reconstruction. Handchir Mikrochir Plast Chir 2002;34(4):251–6.

11. Koshima I, Nanba Y, Takahashi Y, et al. Future of supramicrosurgery as it relates to breast reconstruction: free paraumbilical perforator adiposal flap. Semin Plast Surg 2002;16(1):93–9.

12. Guyuron B. Retroauricular island flap for eye socket reconstruction. Plast Reconstr Surg 1985;76(4):527–33.

13. Song R, Song Y, Qi K, et al. The superior auricular artery and retroauricular arterial island flaps. Plast Reconstr Surg 1996;98(4):657–67.

14. Pinho C, Choupina M, Silva P, et al. A new retroauricular flap for facial reconstruction. Br J Plast Surg 2003;56(6):599–602.

15. Yan D, Tang M, Geddes CR, et al. Vascular anatomy of the integument of the head and neck. In: Blondeel PN, Morris SF, Hallock GG, et al, editors. Perforator flaps. Anatomy, technique, clinical applications. St Louis (MO): Quality Medical Publishing, Inc; 2006. p. 134–60.

16. Boeckx W. Temporoparietal artery perforator flap. In: Blondeel PN, Morris SF, Hallock GG, et al, editors. Perforator flaps. Anatomy, technique, clinical applications. St Louis (MO): Quality Medical Publishing, Inc; 2006. p. 200–15.

17. Özdemir R, Sungur N, Sensöz O, et al. Reconstruction of facial defects with superficial temporal artery island flaps: a donor site with various alternatives. Plast Reconstr Surg 2002;109(5):1528–35.

18. Kilinç H, Bilen BT. A new approach to retroauricular flap transfer: parietal branch-based reverse flow superior auricular artery island flap. Ann Plast Surg 2006;56(4):380–3.

19. Yotsuyanagi T, Watanabe Y, Yamashita K, et al. Retroauricular flap: its clinical application and safety. Br J Plast Surg 2001;54(1):12–9.

20. Kobayashi S, Yoza S, Kakibuchi M, et al. Retroauricular hairline flap transfer to the face. Plast Reconstr Surg 1995;96(1):42–7.

21. Mutter TD. Cases of deformities from burns, relieved by operation. Am J Med Sci 1842;4:66–80.

22. Lamberty BG. The supraclavicular axial patterned flap. Br J Plast Surg 1979;32(3):207–12.

23. Pallua N, Demir E. Postburn head and neck reconstruction in children with the fasciocutaneous supraclavicular artery island flap. Ann Plast Surg 2008; 60(3):276–82.

24. Pallua N, Noah EM. The tunneled supraclavicular island flap: an optimized technique for head and neck reconstruction. Plast Reconstr Surg 2000; 105(3):842–51.

25. Chiu ES, Liu PH, Friedlander PL. Supraclavicular artery island flap for head and neck oncologic reconstruction: indications, complications, and outcomes. Plast Reconstr Surg 2009;124(1):115–23.

26. Cordova A, Pirrello R, D'Arpa S, et al. Vascular anatomy of the supraclavicular area revisited: feasibility of the free supraclavicular perforator flap. Plast Reconstr Surg 2008;122(5):1399–409.

27. Cordova A, D'Arpa S, Pirrello R, et al. Anatomic study on the transverse cervical vessels perforators in the lateral triangle of the neck and harvest of a new flap: the free supraclavicular transverse cervical artery perforator flap. Surg Radiol Anat 2009;31(2):93–100.

28. Hartman EH, Van Damme PA, Sauter H, et al. The use of the pedicled supraclavicular flap in noma reconstructive surgery. J Plast Reconstr Aesthet Surg 2006;59(4):337–42.

29. Spence RJ. An algorithm for total and subtotal facial reconstruction using an expanded transposition flap: a 20-year experience. Plast Reconstr Surg 2008;121(3):795–805.

30. Vesely MJ, Murray DJ, Novak CB, et al. The internal mammary artery perforator flap. An anatomical study and a case report. Ann Plast Surg 2007; 58(2):156–61.

31. Neligan PC, Gullane PJ, Vesely MJ, et al. The internal artery perforator flap: a new variation on an old theme. Plast Reconstr Surg 2007;119(3):891–3.

32. Schmidt M, Aszmann OC, Beck H, et al. The anatomic basis of the internal mammary artery perforator flap: a cadaver study. J Plast Reconstr Aesthet Surg 2008. DOI:10.1016/j.bjps.2008.09.019.

33. Palmer JH, Taylor GI. The vascular territories of the anterior chest wall. Br J Plast Surg 1986;39(3):287–99.

34. Yu P, Roblin P, Chevray P. Internal mammary artery perforator (IMAP) flap for tracheostoma reconstruction. Head Neck 2006;28(8):723–9.

Perforator Flaps in Breast Reconstruction

Charles Y. Tseng, MD, Joan E. Lipa, MD, MSc, FRCS(C)*

KEYWORDS

• DIEP • SIEA • TDAP • SGAP • IGAP • ICAP

A variety of flap designs can be used to create a breast mound that appears and feels similar to the natural breast. The trend in breast cancer treatment is toward less deforming methods to excise the tumor while sparing normal surrounding tissue. The development of perforator flaps parallels this trend in that current techniques have evolved toward the harvest of autologous tissue with minimal disruption of the muscle through which the blood vessels pass. The evolution of workhorse flaps such as the free transverse rectus abdominis myocutaneous (free-TRAM) flap into the muscle sparing-TRAM (MS-TRAM) and deep inferior epigastric artery perforator (DIEP) flap variations highlights this trend toward lower donor site morbidity.

A variety of methods have been used to name and describe perforator flaps, including anatomic location and arterial supply. In the absence of a standardized naming scheme for these flaps, multiple names for the same flap proliferated in the literature, resulting in confusion and misunderstanding. With the Gent consensus, however, it is now standard to name a perforator flap according to its artery of origin.[1] Anatomic studies show that the parent artery to a perforator flap commonly arises on the deep surface of the muscle and gives off musculocutaneous perforating vessels that penetrate through the muscle to supply the overlying fat and skin. In other instances, a vessel may branch off the parent artery and travel through a septocutaneous membrane to the skin paddle. These vessels are referred to as septocutaneous perforator vessels.

Careful, meticulous dissection of the perforating vessels down through the muscles to the parent artery yields the purest form of a perforator flap and thereby preserves the entire muscle along with its motor nerves. Occasionally, anatomic variation or concerns about tissue perfusion encountered intraoperatively may guide the decision to include some muscle in the flap, thereby changing the design of the flap to one of its muscle-sparing variants.

The psychological power of immediate breast reconstruction combined with the bonus of an abdominoplasty or buttock lift appeals to many patients. However, not all patients are candidates for immediate reconstruction, and not all women opt for mastectomy. Some women may require delayed reconstruction or partial reconstruction of breast-conserving deformities. In addition, the paucity of lower abdominal tissue or previous abdominal surgery, such as cosmetic abdominoplasty, liposuction, laparotomy, or previous pedicled TRAM reconstruction may preclude using the lower abdominal tissues for reconstruction. These contraindications coupled with the need for alternative options for autologous breast reconstruction drive the search for new donor sites and the development of new flap designs.

LOWER ABDOMINAL FLAPS

Flap designs for the lower abdominal donor site highlight the evolution and sophistication of microsurgical technique. Hartrampf's introduction of the pedicled TRAM flap in 1982 ushered in the modern era of breast reconstruction. Further investigation into the vascular anatomy of this flap design revealed that the dominant arterial supply to the rectus abdominis muscle is the deep inferior epigastric artery (DIEA).[2,3] Understanding that the rectus abdominis muscle can carry a larger subcutaneous fat and skin paddle when based on the

Division of Plastic and Reconstructive Surgery, David Geffen School of Medicine, University of California Los Angeles, 200 UCLA Medical Plaza, Suite 465, Los Angeles, CA 90095, USA
* Corresponding author.
E-mail address: jlipa@mednet.ucla.edu

Clin Plastic Surg 37 (2010) 641–654
doi:10.1016/j.cps.2010.06.002

deep system, many microsurgeons adopted the free-TRAM flap for breast reconstruction.

For many reconstructive surgeons, it became clear that donor site morbidity could be lowered by reducing the amount of muscle taken with the flap and injury to the muscle left behind. The concepts of donor site muscle sparing were introduced with the segmental latissimus dorsi myocutaneous and free-TRAM flaps.[4,5] Koshima[6] refined this concept even further when he used the skin paddle overlying the rectus abdominis muscle for reconstruction of the mouth and groin. Koshima's flap designs were based on a single paraumbilical perforating vessel off the DIEA and composed of subcutaneous fat and skin only. Soon after, Allen performed the first deep inferior epigastric perforator (DIEP) flap for breast reconstruction by transferring the lower abdominal fat and skin of a TRAM flap while sparing the underlying rectus abdominis muscle.[7]

Whereas pedicled TRAM and free-TRAM flaps remain workhorses, the quest to minimize donor site morbidity has given rise to the development of the MS-TRAM and DIEP flap designs, each of which spare more muscle. Nahabedian and colleagues[8] developed a classification system to describe the degree of sparing of the rectus abdominis muscle: MS-0 describes the sacrifice of the full-width (partial length) of the muscle; MS-1 describes the preservation of the lateral segment; MS-2 describes the preservation of the lateral and medial segments; and MS-3 refers to the preservation of all the rectus muscle (the equivalent of a DIEP flap).

This classification system shows the continuum that exists among these flaps, which require the disruption of the anterior rectus sheath and variable amounts of rectus abdominis muscle.[9] Hence, the primary advantage of a perforator flap is that it spares the underlying muscle and motor innervation, thereby reducing morbidity and preserving functionality.

Distinct from these flaps is the superficial inferior epigastric artery (SIEA) flap, which was first described by Grotting in 1991 and termed the free abdominoplasty flap.[10] This design precludes dissection below the rectus sheath because the superficial epigastric artery and vein arise from the femoral vessels and head directly into the subcutaneous fat of the lower abdomen.

DIEP Flaps

Most women with breast cancer who have or have had mastectomy are potential candidates for DIEP flap breast reconstruction and will be of an age where they have excess fat and skin overlying the lower abdomen. The fat in this region is typically soft and easy to shape and therefore most closely approximates the feel of a normal breast. In most cases, and even for most thin patients, the tissue found in the lower abdominal region is sufficient to reconstruct a breast mound. In an 8-year review of 172 patients who underwent breast reconstruction with tissue from the lower abdomen, Granzow and colleagues[11] found that the weight of the harvested flaps averaged approximately 120% of the weight of the mastectomy specimens in immediate reconstructions. Thus, the harvested flap is often trimmed of excess tissue and thin patients (who tend to have smaller breast volumes to replace) often have enough lower abdominal tissue to closely match the contralateral breast.

An absolute contraindication specific to the use of the lower abdominal tissues for breast reconstruction is previous abdominoplasty. Previous abdominal liposuction does not preclude DIEP flap elevation,[12] but caution should be exercised to ensure proper preoperative and intraoperative perforator evaluation before committing to elevating the abdominal tissue as a DIEP flap in this situation. Active smoking within 4 to 6 weeks of planned surgery contributes to fat necrosis/partial flap loss, delayed wound healing, and random flap loss at both the mastectomy and abdominal donor sites.

Previous abdominal surgery through incisions that traverse the desired skin paddle can also affect the design of the flap reconstruction. For example, the subcutaneous fat and skin lateral to an appendectomy scar may not adequately perfuse after flap elevation. Similarly, the skin paddle contralateral to a midline abdominal scar may not perfuse well enough after flap elevation to survive transfer to the breast. However, each hemiflap could be viable if elevated on its own DIEA or SIEA pedicle.

Patients are also encouraged to complete any radiation therapy to the chest before surgical breast reconstruction. Although the perforator flaps usually tolerate radiation well, a superior long-term result is typically obtained in reconstructions performed after rather than before chest wall radiation. This strategy spares the flap from the damaging effects of radiation and allows the removal of thick, stiff irradiated chest wall skin. It is then replaced with soft, nonradiated abdominal skin and soft tissue.[13]

Excellent state-of-the-art descriptions of DIEP flap elevation have been published; the reader is directed to these articles for detailed description of technique.[9,11,14,15]

For all flaps, a fusiform ellipse is outlined on the lower abdomen that extends from the suprapubic crease inferiorly to just above the umbilicus superiorly and laterally to the anterior superior iliac spine. However, the amount of tissue that can be safely taken and still allow for closure of the donor site must be estimated.[9] The surgeon must also estimate how much of the lower abdominal flap is required to provide the volume necessary for appropriate reconstruction of the breast. For unilateral DIEP flap reconstruction, Zones 1 to 3 can be reliably transferred on a single adequately sized perforator from the medial row and zone 4 is typically removed.[16] An adequate perforator should have a vein greater than 1 mm in diameter where it enters the flap and a palpable or visibly pulsating artery.[17] The portion of the flap that is used for breast reconstruction should be centered on the dominant perforator to provide the best flap perfusion and to avoid fat necrosis (**Fig. 1**).[14] In the situation in which the entire lower abdominal flap is desired or needed to match the large contralateral breast, the contralateral deep inferior epigastric (DIE) pedicle, a perforator from the contralateral hemiflap, or the contralateral superficial system pedicle can be anastomosed to the side branch of the main ipsilateral pedicle, thereby creating a supercharged or turbocharged construct (**Fig. 2**).[18,19]

In bilateral reconstruction, the transverse skin paddle is usually split down the midline, yielding two hemiflaps, each with its own vascular pedicle. Thus, the DIEP flap design is ideal for bilateral reconstruction as complete muscle-sparing, and preservation of the motor nerves to each rectus abdominis muscle significantly reduces donor site morbidity relative to free-TRAM and MS-TRAM flap designs.

The DIEP flap has proven reliability and a low complication rate. In their experience, Allen and colleagues[11] reported that 25% of flaps were based on one perforator, 50% on 2 perforators,

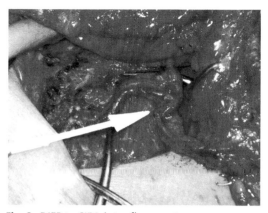

Fig. 2. DIEP to SIEA intra-flap anastomoses.

and 25% on 3 or more perforators. In a 10-year retrospective review of 758 DIEP flaps by the same group,[20] 6% of patients returned to the operating room for flap-related problems. Partial flap loss occurred in 2.5% of cases. Total flap loss occurred in less than 1% of all cases. Problems with the vein or venous anastomoses were nearly 8 times more likely than problems with the artery or arterial anastomoses. Fat necrosis appeared in 13% of flaps. Seroma formation at the abdominal donor site was approximately 5%. Abdominal hernia occurred in 0.7% of cases.

Nahabedian and colleagues[21] reported their experience with the MS-2 TRAM and DIEP flaps. For MS-2 TRAM flaps, the complications included total necrosis in 1.8% of cases, fat necrosis in 7.1%, venous congestion in 2.7%, and abdominal bulge in 4.6% of unilateral reconstruction and 21% of bilateral reconstruction. In comparison, the DIEP flap group complications included total necrosis in 2.7% of cases, fat necrosis in 6.4%, venous congestion in 4.5%, and abdominal bulge rates of 1.5% after unilateral reconstruction and 4.5% after bilateral reconstruction.

SIEA Flaps

Although not a true perforator flap in the sense that the SIEA does not give off vessels that penetrate through muscle or traverse through a septum to supply overlying fat and skin, harvest of an SIEA flap precludes the need to open the anterior rectus sheath. Thus, breast reconstruction using the SIEA flap virtually eliminates donor site morbidity when compared with DIEP flap harvest. There is no risk of a new abdominal hernia and even less abdominal pain compared with other abdominal flaps that require disruption of the anterior rectus sheath.

Despite these compelling advantages, several factors should be considered before SIEA flap

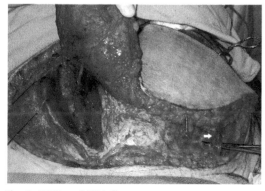

Fig. 1. DIEP and SIEA flaps.

breast reconstruction is performed. First, the SIEA flap is limited by variability in its vascular anatomy and skin territory. The SIEA and vein are inconsistently present, or of sufficient caliber, to reliably perfuse the volume of tissue needed for breast reconstruction. The SIEA is absent in approximately 35% to 51% of the population and not suitable, mainly because of small diameter, in an additional 19% of cases.[2,22] Compared with the DIEA (2–4 mm), the superficial artery is typically smaller (mean diameter 1.1–1.6 mm), has a shorter pedicle length (mean 7 cm), and can be size-mismatched when anastomosed to the thoracodorsal or internal mammary artery recipients. If present and being considered for use, it should be of sufficient caliber with a minimum external diameter of at least 1.5 mm at the level of the lower abdominal incision where it enters the flap, and have a palpable or visible pulse.[22,23] Because the superficial vessels are more lateral than the lateral row of rectus abdominis perforators and because they enter into the edge of the flap, insetting in the chest may be more difficult compared with the DIEP flap and the artery should be transected just distal to its takeoff from the femoral artery to ensure adequate pedicle length.

Thus, the pitfalls of the SIEA flap design are the inconsistent vascular anatomy, the shorter and smaller-caliber arterial pedicle, and the inconsistent perfusion/drainage across the midline. Some surgeons believe that the amount of skin and fat that may be safely carried by an SIEA flap is limited to zones 1 and 2, and any tissue taken more than 1 to 2 cm past the midline demarcates and necroses after the initial reconstruction.[24] In contrast, some have been able to successfully harvest tissue across the midline as long as zone 4 and any poorly perfused tissues are excised after the completion of the anastomosis.[23] Recent intraoperative perfusion studies using laser-fluorescence-videoangiography have clearly shown that perfusion beyond the midline was unreliable and that the contralateral hemiflap should be discarded.[25]

When the harvested SIEA flaps were based on arteries with diameters 1.5 mm or greater, reported complication rates included fat necrosis (3.7%), partial flap loss (3.7%), arterial thrombosis (3.7%), and venous congestion (3.7%). In contrast, when the harvested SIEA flaps included arteries with diameters less than 1.5 mm, reported complication rates included arterial thrombosis (8.3%), total flap loss (6.9%), partial flap loss (5.6%), and venous congestion (1.4%). As would be expected, there were no complications with abdominal bulge or hernia.[23]

With these considerations in mind, the SIEA flap is ideal for reconstruction of small to medium-sized breasts using a hemiflap. It is particularly advantageous in bilateral breast reconstruction. Even if only one of the hemiflaps is of the SIEA design, the abdominal donor site is effectively converted into a unilateral MS-TRAM or DIEP flap donor site. This strategy avoids the need for a bilateral MS-TRAM or DIEP flap donor site, which are associated with more morbidity in terms of effects on abdominal strength and contour compared with unilateral TRAM and DIEP donor sites.

As clinical and scientific evidence emerges, it becomes evident that the SIEA flap does not represent a substitution for flap designs based on the deep inferior epigastric system. Rather, it should be considered an alternative in well-selected patients to achieve breast reconstruction of equal aesthetic quality and decrease abdominal donor site morbidity. Typical parameters for DIEP and SIEA flaps are found in **Table 1**.

GLUTEAL ARTERY PERFORATOR FLAPS

Of those patients who seek autogenous breast reconstruction, driving factors range from the simple preference for the concept of autologous tissue reconstruction and complementary body contouring to the more complex safety concerns surrounding implants in the setting of previous chest wall radiation therapy. Nonetheless, not all are candidates for reconstruction using tissues from the lower abdomen. This situation continues to push the development and inclusion of other donor sites into the microsurgeon's armamentarium.

Just as the DIEP flap naturally evolved from the free-TRAM and MS-TRAM predecessors, the superior gluteal artery perforator (SGAP) and inferior gluteal artery perforator (IGAP) flaps have evolved from the superiorly or inferiorly based free gluteal myocutaneous flap.

Terminal branches of the internal iliac artery, the superior and inferior gluteal arteries pass out of the pelvis above and below the piriformis muscle to supply the upper and lower halves of the gluteus maximus muscle, respectively. As the superior gluteal artery passes through the greater sciatic foramen, it divides into a superficial and a deep branch. The superficial branch supplies the gluteus muscle and sends perforating vessels that penetrate the muscle to supply the overlying subcutaneous fat and skin of the upper buttock. The inferior gluteal artery accompanies the greater sciatic nerve, the internal pudendal vessels, and the posterior

Table 1
DIEP and SIEA flap parameters

Parameter	DIEP Flap Vessels		SIEA Flap Vessels	
	Average	Range	Average	Range
Pedicle length (cm)	8–10	Up to 20.5	7	Up to 15
DIE artery diameter (mm)		2–3	1.4	0.8–1.8
DIE vein diameter (mm)		2–3.5	>2	

femoral cutaneous nerve. It exits the pelvis caudal to the piriformis muscle and travels under the inferior portion of the gluteus maximus, giving off perforating vessels that penetrate the muscle to supply the overlying fat and skin of the lower buttock.[26]

Perforating vessels closer to the medial aspect of the buttock have short intramuscular lengths, whereas those located laterally must travel more obliquely through the muscle substance. Therefore, pedicles based on perforators to the lateral aspects of the skin paddle tend to be longer than those based on medial perforators. When compared with the course of the superior gluteal vessels, the course of the inferior gluteal vessels is more oblique through the gluteus maximus muscle. Hence, the IGAP pedicle has the potential to be longer than the SGAP pedicle.[24] More importantly, the superior inferior and inferior gluteal arteries and veins should be carefully dissected down to their takeoff from the internal iliac vessels to obtain adequate size match with the recipient internal mammary artery and vein (average diameter = 2.5–3.5 mm) (**Figs. 3** and **4**).

Indications

These flaps are generally considered a second-line option after the DIEP flap for autologous breast reconstruction. Patients ideally suited for GAP breast reconstruction include women without sufficient abdominal tissue, those with a history of previous abdominal surgery, or those who have more subcutaneous tissue in the buttock region than in the abdominal region (**Figs. 5** and **6**). In addition, the younger patient with genetic risk factors predisposing to breast cancer who elects prophylactic mastectomy may lack sufficient abdominal tissue for bilateral reconstruction but usually has enough tissue in the buttock region for immediate or staged bilateral GAP flap reconstruction.

General advantages of GAP flap reconstruction include an associated body contouring procedure (modest buttock lift) at the same time as breast reconstruction, and a shorter scar that can be well concealed by clothing or camouflaged in the natural body contours. However, the skin paddle is designed to be longer than it is wide and may be inadequately sized if a large area of skin replacement is needed, as might be required in

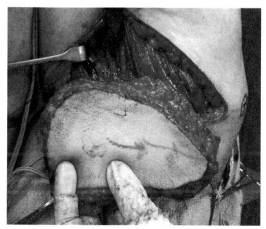

Fig. 3. IGAP flap with long pedicle.

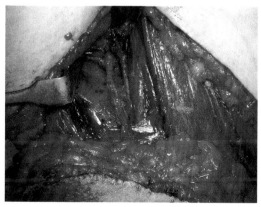

Fig. 4. Close-up view of IGAP flap pedicle dissection to internal iliac vessels.

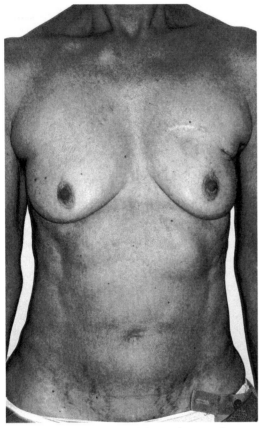

Fig. 5. Insufficient lower abdominal tissue for DIEP flap.

delayed reconstruction after chest wall radiation therapy.

Unlike the soft and pliable tissues of the lower abdominal region, the gluteal subcutaneous fat is globular and supported by dense fibrous septa, making it firmer when compared with abdominal

fat. This characteristic gives it good projection for the limited volume of tissue harvested but also makes it more difficult to shape into a breast mound (**Fig. 7**). Patients undergoing unilateral reconstruction with GAP flaps may require secondary procedures such as fat grafting and liposuction to achieve symmetry and satisfactory breast shape. More significant disadvantages include a high risk of seroma formation and a relative contour deformity of the unilateral buttock donor site such that many patients request secondary buttock symmetry procedures as well.

Absolute contraindications include previous gluteal surgery or buttock lift involving the donor site and active smoking. Relative contraindications include previous cosmetic liposuction of the gluteal donor site because of possible injury to the perforators. Caution should be exercised with proper preoperative radiologic imaging and intraoperative perforator evaluation.[12]

SGAP Flaps

The superior gluteal artery myocutaneous flap has been used for autologous breast reconstruction but is associated with a difficult dissection and a short pedicle such that interposition vein grafts were often needed to reach the intended recipient vessels.[27] In 1995, Allen and Tucker[28] described the SGAP flap for breast reconstruction. Dissection of the perforating vessels out of the muscle yielded two key advantages compared with the original myocutaneous predecessor. Specifically, dissection of the perforator vessels out of the muscle made dissection of the superior gluteal artery easier and, perhaps more importantly, resulted in a longer pedicle such that microvascular transfer can be completed without the need for

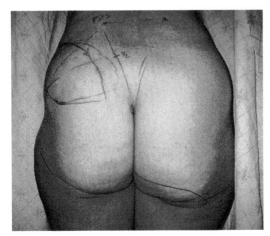

Fig. 6. Buttock donor site.

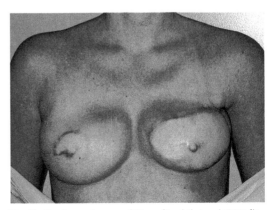

Fig. 7. Contour abnormalities after bilateral GAP flap reconstruction.

interposition vein grafting. Like the DIEP flap, no sacrifice of muscle is required.

Excellent state-of-the-art descriptions of SGAP and IGAP flap elevation have been published; the reader is directed to these articles.[28,29]

Based on their 9-year experience with 142 GAP flaps, Allen and colleagues[26] suggest basing the flap on a single large perforator, if present, and adjusting the orientation of the typical oblique, superomedial-to-inferolateral skin paddle to a more horizontal design to reduce postoperative contour deformity and thereby place the scar in a more favorable position. These investigators also suggest using perforators positioned laterally on the long axis of the flap to maximize pedicle length. Furthermore, the internal mammary vessels are the preferred recipients given the shorter pedicle length of the SGAP flap. Typical SGAP flap parameters are found in **Table 2**.

Reported complications included arterial and venous complication (6%), donor site contour deformity requiring secondary correction (4%), partial flap necrosis (4%), donor site seroma (2%), and donor site hematoma (1%).[26]

IGAP Flaps

Early experience with the inferior gluteal myocutaneous flap and IGAP flap used an oblique, superolateral-to-inferomedial skin paddle. The literature describes significant donor site morbidity associated with this flap design. The most significant problems were postoperative lower extremity dysesthesia and pain syndromes.[30,31]

Modification of the skin paddle design to a more horizontal skin paddle located just above and parallel to the gluteal crease resulted in a significant improvement in donor site morbidity (**Fig. 8**). The flap is elevated in the subfascial plane and the perforators approached from lateral to medial. A single large perforator is typically used but multiple perforators in the same plane of muscle-splitting dissection can be incorporated into the flap. Limiting dissection over the sciatic nerve precludes sciatic nerve exposure, and leaving a sufficient fat pad medially over the ischium reduces postoperative pain syndromes. The scar is hidden in the gluteal crease (**Fig. 9**).

PEDICLED PERFORATOR FLAPS

Used in conjunction with prosthetic devices or on its own, the pedicled latissimus dorsi myocutaneous flap is a reliable workhorse for breast reconstruction with autogenous tissue. The application of perforator principles to this workhorse is a logical extension of its design and dramatically broadens the range of applications and decreases donor site morbidity. Angrigiani and colleagues[32] were the first to describe harvesting the cutaneous island of the latissimus dorsi flap without muscle. They based the flap on one perforator and transferred the tissue as a free flap or transposed it as a pedicled flap.

In comparison, the intercostal artery myocutaneous flap has also been well described[33] but has found limited use in reconstructive breast surgery, likely as a result of pain and contour deformities at the donor site. The application of perforator principles to this flap has greatly expanded the range of options available to the reconstructive surgeon asked to correct the partial

Table 2
SGAP and IGAP flap parameters

Parameter	SGAP Flaps		IGAP Flap	
	Average	Range	Average	Range
Size				
Width (cm)	9.5	7–12	8	7–10
Length (cm)	24.5	16–29	18	15–22
Approximate weight (g)	451	190–894	425	148–833
Vessels				
Pedicle length (cm)	9.1	7–12		8–11
Gluteal artery diameter (mm)	3.38	2–4.5	>2	2–4.5
Gluteal vein diameter (mm)	3.9	2.5–4.5	3.5	3–4

Data from Holm C, Mayr M, Hofter E, et al. The versatility of the SIEA flap: a clinical assessment of the vascular territory of the superficial epigastric inferior artery. J Plast Reconstr Aesthet Surg 2007;60:946–51; and Allen RJ, Tucker C. Superior gluteal artery perforator free flap for breast reconstruction. Plast Reconstr Surg 1995;95:1207–12.

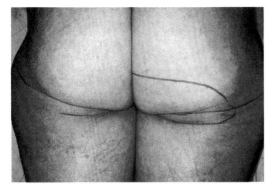

Fig. 8. IGAP flap design in the crease.

mastectomy defect and restore breast contour with a sensate flap. Variations of the intercostal artery perforator (ICAP) flap will become workhorses as surgeons become more familiar with its design and applications.

Therefore, patients with breast or thoracic defects amenable to latissimus dorsi myoocutaneous or intercostal artery myocutaneous flap reconstruction are also ideal candidates for reconstruction with pedicled perforator flaps. These flaps may also be transferred to distant sites as free flaps, if needed.

Thoracodorsal Artery Perforator Flaps

As the thoracodorsal artery passes beneath the latissimus dorsi muscle, it gives off the serratus anterior artery branch and splits into a transverse and vertical branch just before entering the muscle. From these branches, numerous perforating vessels of various size penetrate the muscle to supply the overlying subcutaneous fat and skin.

Adequately sized perforators for inclusion in a perforator flap are those that are greater than 0.5 mm in diameter. These perforators are usually found on the proximal portions of the transverse and vertical branches closer to the hilus. In relation to surface landmarks, this is within 7 to 10 cm distal to the posterior axillary fold and within 5 cm of the anterior border of the latissimus muscle.[34] The vertical branch gives off an average of 1.8 perforators (range 1–4) and the transverse branch gives off an average of 1.4 perforators (range 1–3).

Anatomic studies have also identified an inconsistent direct cutaneous branch off the extramuscular portion of the thoracodorsal artery in 55% of cases.[35] This direct cutaneous branch takes off proximal to the vascular hilus and courses around the anterior border of the muscle to supply the overlying fat and skin. Thus, the thoracodorsal artery perforator (TDAP) flap can be based on either the penetrating musculocutaneous or direct cutaneous perforators.

In regards to flap design, an ellipse centered over the free upper or preferably lateral border of the latissimus dorsi muscle captures the perforators coming off the transverse or vertical branch of the thoracodorsal artery, respectively (**Fig. 10**). Care should be taken to locate the skin paddle near the neurovascular hilus because the desired perforators are found on the proximal segments of the transverse and vertical branch. In relation to surface landmarks, the neurovascular hilus

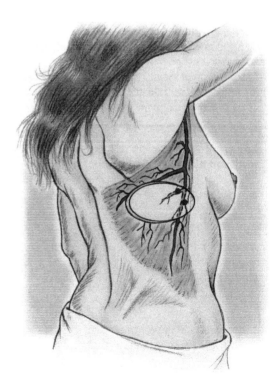

Fig. 10. TDAP flap.

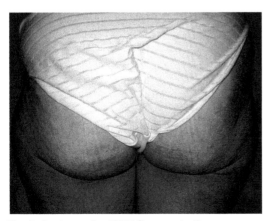

Fig. 9. Postoperative IGAP flap scar in the crease.

can be located approximately 3 to 6 cm distal to the inferior scapular border and 1 to 4 cm posterior to the anterior border of the latissimus dorsi muscle.[35] Given these anatomic findings, a multitude of flap designs can be used so long as an adequately sized perforator is included. Typical TDAP flap parameters are found in **Table 3**.

Like its myocutaneous predecessor, the TDAP flap is well suited for immediate or delayed partial breast reconstruction, correction of breast deformities after lumpectomy, and as a salvage procedure for partial loss of a previous flap. The TDAP flap can also be used in conjunction with prosthetic devices and to resurface or replace skin as needed. Given its arc of rotation, the TDAP flap can be transposed into the superolateral, inferolateral, and inferomedial quadrants of the breast. Although there are few contraindications to perforator flap reconstruction, injury to the thoracodorsal pedicle from previous axillary or thoracic surgery is an absolute contraindication. Experience with perforator flap techniques is recommended.

An excellent description of the surgical technique has been published.[36] The main points are highlighted herein. To anticipate the presence of the direct cutaneous perforator, the anterior border of the skin paddle should lie in front of the anterior border of the latissimus dorsi muscle. Depending on the indication and desired arc of rotation, the flap is planned as a vertical or horizontal ellipse over the latissimus dorsi muscle. The selected perforator should be large (>0.5 mm) and visibly pulsatile. Once a suitable perforator is identified, the cleavage plane of the latissimus dorsi muscle in which the perforator resides is developed and dissection continues down to the thoracodorsal artery (**Fig. 11**). The main thoracodorsal pedicle is dissected free until the desired pedicle length is obtained. The flap is then pulled

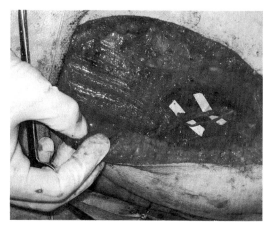

Fig. 11. TDAP pedicle dissection.

through the muscle and transposed into the defect.

Like the DIEP flap, conversion to a muscle-sparing design is warranted for a variety of situations. Muscle-sparing latissimus dorsi (MS-LD) flaps are defined as: MS-LD 1, in which a 2 × 4 cm segment of muscle is incorporated around the perforators; MS-LD 2, in which a segment up to 5 cm in width is incorporated in the flap; and MS-LD 3, in which most of the muscle is included in the flap. When the perforators are small (<0.5 mm) but pulsatile or are separated by a thin strip of muscle, conversion to an MS-LD 1 increases safety by preserving a cuff muscle to reduce the risk of perforator rupture or avulsion. When the perforators are smaller than 0.5 mm and nonpulsatile, the flap should be converted to an MS-LD 2 and thereby incorporate a maximum number of perforators.[36]

ICAP Flaps

The ICAP flap is based on the same intercostal neurovascular pedicle of the more familiar intercostal myocutaneous flaps. Whereas the standard intercostal myocutaneous flap includes harvest of the intercostal muscles, application of perforator flap techniques allows the surgeon to transpose the desired skin paddle and preserve the associated musculature. Compared with other perforator flaps for breast reconstruction, a unique advantage of the ICAP flaps is that these pedicle perforator flaps can be transposed as sensate flaps by including the associated intercostal nerve.

For the purposes of breast reconstruction, Hamdi and colleagues[37] have described the lateral ICAP (LICAP) flap and the anterior ICAP (AICAP) flap based on the posterior intercostal artery and the anterior intercostal artery, respectively. Indications include immediate or delayed partial breast

Parameter	TDAP Flaps	
	Average (cm)	Range (cm)
Size		
Width	8	6–10
Length	20	16–25
Perforator location		
Distal to posterior axillary fold	10.8	8–13
Anterior border of LD	2.8	0–5

Table 3
TDAP flap parameters

reconstruction, salvage after partial flap necrosis, and postmastectomy breast reconstruction in combination with expander or implant. The LICAP flap has also been used for autologous breast augmentation in the massive weight loss population and for correction of congenital asymmetry.[38,39] Contraindications to ICAP flap harvest include previous thoracotomy or radiation therapy to the chest wall that may have also injured the perforator vessels.

The anatomy and course of the intercostal vessels have been extensively studied and described. The posterior intercostal vessels communicate with the anterior intercostal vessels to create a vascular arcade between the aorta and internal mammary vessels.[33,40] Perforating vessels from the posterior intercostal artery penetrate the intercostal musculature to supply the overlying subcutaneous fat and skin. Similarly, perforators from the internal mammary artery and the anterior intercostal vessels supply the pectoralis major muscle and overlying skin. Thus, a subcutaneous fat and skin paddle centered over one of these perforators can be designed, harvested, and transposed to cover defects of the breast, chest, and thorax (**Fig. 12**).

In the intercostal segment, the intercostal neurovascular bundle lies deep to the external and internal intercostal muscles and superficial to the innermost intercostal muscle. This segment is particularly useful because the artery gives off between 5 and 7 musculocutaneous perforators at intervals of 1 to 3 cm. The major perforators are approximately 0.8 mm in diameter. At the midaxillary line, the posterior intercostal artery gives off a lateral cutaneous branch that passes just anterior to the anterior border of the latissimus dorsi muscle to supply the overlying skin. Hamdi and colleagues[41] recently published a detailed anatomic study of the lateral intercostal

perforators. A mean value of 3.91 perforators per side was found. Most of the intercostal perforators were found between the fifth and the eighth intercostal space level (88.4%). Mean distances of intercostal perforators to the anterior border of the latissimus dorsi muscle varied between 2.67 and 3.49 cm. The largest or dominant perforator was most frequently found in the sixth intercostal space (38.6% of cases) at an average of 2.5 to 3.5 cm from the anterior border of the latissimus dorsi muscle.

The reader is referred to excellent detailed descriptions of surgical technique.[37] Typical ICAP flap parameters are found in **Table 4**. The LICAP flap is based on the lateral cutaneous branch or other perforators from the intercostal segment of the posterior intercostal artery that pierce the serratus anterior. These perforators are located anterior to the latissimus dorsi muscle. Anatomic studies suggest that LICAP flaps up to 25 × 20 cm can be raised. However, the maximum width that can be closed primarily is less than 12 cm. The posterior border of the flap should lie at least 5 cm behind the posterior axillary line to ensure capture of the lateral cutaneous branch of the posterior intercostal artery (**Fig. 13**). The posterior border of the flap is incised and elevated off the underlying latissimus muscle until reaching its anterior border. Once an adequately sized perforator is identified and preserved, dissection follows the perforator vessel to its parent vessel, carefully splitting the surrounding muscle along fibers. A pedicle length of 3 to 5 cm is adequate to reach a defect of the superior, inferior, and lateral parts of the breast. If a longer pedicle is required, dissection of the main pedicle can continue on within the costal groove.

The AICAP flap is based on a perforator of the anterior intercostal artery typically located 1 to 3 cm lateral to the sternal edge.[37] The perforator is located using a pencil Doppler and the flap designed around the perforator. The flap is elevated from lateral to medial and from caudal to cranial. The appropriate perforator is identified and preserved. Depending on the location of the perforator, the pectoralis or rectus abdominis muscle is split and dissection of the perforator continues down toward the parent anterior intercostal or internal mammary artery. The AICAP flap is primarily used for reconstruction of partial superomedial, and inferomedial breast defects.

PREOPERATIVE IMAGING

As described above, there are many options for perforator flap reconstruction of the breast. Before the era of preoperative imaging, a surgeon had

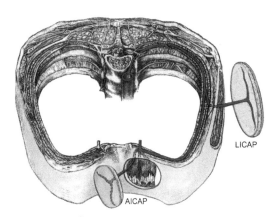

Fig. 12. ICAP flaps.

Table 4
LICAP and AICAP flap parameters

Parameter	LICAP Flaps		AICAP Flaps	
	Average (cm)	Range (cm)	Average (cm)	Range (cm)
Size				
Width	Up to 12 (for primary closure)	Up to 20	8	7–10
Length	24.5	Up to 25	18	

only general anatomic knowledge of perforator anatomy. Patient-specific anatomy could be obtained only after surgery was well under way. As a result, the process of perforator vessel selection could become tedious, worrisome, and often lengthened the overall operative time. The increasing use of perforator flaps escalates the need for preoperative familiarity with a patient's anatomic features, particularly as it pertains to the surgical anatomy and course of the desired perforator to its parent vessel. Assessment of perforators to aid in preoperative planning became routine with the widespread use of noninvasive preoperative imaging modalities such as duplex ultrasonography and color duplex sonography. More recent advances in computed tomography (CT) and magnetic resonance (MR) imaging have revolutionized the planning process.

Although portable and simple to use, unidirectional hand-held Doppler ultrasound cannot differentiate perforating vessels from superficial and deep axial vessels or robust perforator vessels from small ones. It also cannot accurately locate perforators that do not exit perpendicular from the fascia and cannot provide data about the anatomic course of a vessel.[42] Duplex ultrasonography and color duplex sonography have been used but significant inconsistencies between the imaging results and operative findings are common, likely because of the requirement of experienced technicians with knowledge of perforator anatomy. Furthermore, the resolution of the sonographic modalities is limited and the presentation of the imaged data is somewhat counterintuitive to the three-dimensional nature of surgery.

On the other hand, computed tomographic angiography (CTA) is a new technique that provides detailed information about vascular anatomy as well as soft and bony tissue without the risks of traditional angiography. More importantly, reformatting the information into three-dimensional images uniquely shows anatomic relationships among blood vessels, bones, and soft tissue.

CTA is shown to be an effective tool for mapping the arterial and venous circulation to various body regions, including the head and lower limbs.[43] Standard imaging protocols have been described and published studies report a high sensitivity of CTA data to operative findings. Rozen and colleagues[44,45] found that CTA was superior to Doppler ultrasound for preoperative assessment of the vascular supply to the lower abdominal donor site for DIEA perforator flaps. CTA was superior at identifying the location and course of the perforator vessels, facilitated intraoperative decision making, reduced surgical error in identification of perforator anatomy, and reduced operative times. In addition, the wealth of information obtained after CTA imaging can be used to direct the surgeon to the most successful operative plan (**Figs. 14** and **15**). This factor is particularly applicable in those patients who have had

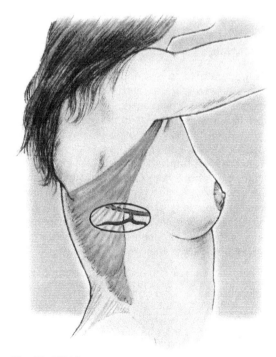

Fig. 13. LICAP.

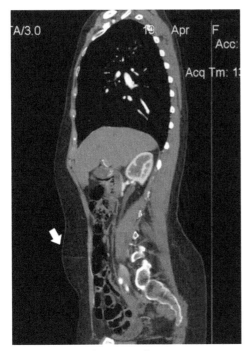

Fig. 14. CTA sagittal view: perforator.

previous abdominal or gluteal liposuction and desire DIEP or GAP flap breast reconstruction.[12] Thus, CTA accuracy in perforator mapping can directly influence the decision to operate and guide the surgeon toward the operation to perform.[46]

Although CTA has effectively become the gold standard in preoperative imaging and planning for perforator flap surgery, there are concerns about the potential hazards of ionizing radiation and nephrotoxic contrast administration. In contrast, MR imaging precludes exposure to ionizing radiation. Recent advances in MR

technology have improved the spatial resolution of small-caliber vessels such that 1-mm perforating vessels can be detected. Furthermore, gadolinium-containing contrast agents used in MR angiography (MRA) have a lower incidence of acute allergic reaction compared with iodinated contrast used in CTA (0.07% vs 3%). Nonetheless, gadolinium can potentially induce nephrogenic systemic fibrosis. This is a rare disease, with just more than 200 cases reported worldwide in patients with impaired renal function.[46] Creatinine levels should be checked before MRA in patients with a history of renal disease, hypertension, diabetes, or other disease that impairs renal function. CTA should also be considered in those patients who cannot undergo MRA because of metal implants or claustrophobia.

Early experience with MRA shows that it is a reliable preoperative imaging technique for breast reconstruction with abdominal perforator flaps and gluteal perforator flaps. Like CTA, MRA data can be reformatted in a variety of anatomic planes and three-dimensional perspectives easily interpreted by the operating surgeon. MRA provides exceptional anatomic details to accurately evaluate the arborization pattern of a vessel in the subcutaneous fat, map the location at which perforators penetrate the fascia, determine relative vessel size, and show the course traveled by the vessel.[47–49] This kind of detailed preoperative information allows the surgeon to select the optimal perforator and center the flap around it, shorten operative times, and improve outcomes.

SUMMARY

The perforator flaps described above can be used to recreate a durable and naturally appearing breast mound. The variety of perforator flaps from donor sites that include the trunk, abdomen, and buttock can be transposed as pedicled or free flaps for partial or complete breast reconstruction. Preoperative CT and MR imaging provide detailed information about vascular anatomy in relation to soft and bony tissues without the risks of traditional angiography. This information can guide the surgeon toward the most successful operative plan, particularly in patients who have undergone previous surgery of the desired donor site.

REFERENCES

1. Blondeel PN, Van Landuyt KH, Monstrey SJ, et al. The "Gent" consensus on perforator flap terminology: preliminary definitions. Plast Reconstr Surg 2003;112:1378–83.

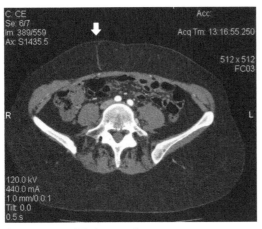

Fig. 15. CTA axial view: perforator.

2. Taylor GI, Daniel RK. The anatomy of several free flap donor sites. Plast Reconstr Surg 1975;56: 243–53.

3. Boyd JB, Taylor GI, Corlett R. The vascular territories of the superior epigastric and the deep inferior epigastric systems. Plast Reconstr Surg 1984;73: 1–14.

4. Elliott LF, Raffel B, Wade J. Segmental latissimus dorsi free flap: clinical considerations. Ann Plast Surg 1989;23:231–8.

5. Feller AM. Free TRAM. Results and abdominal wall function. Clin Plast Surg 1994;21:232.

6. Koshima I, Moriguchi T, Soeda S, et al. Free thin paraumbilical perforator-based flaps. Ann Plast Surg 1994;32:12–7.

7. Allen RJ, Treece P. Deep inferior epigastric perforator flap for breast reconstruction. Ann Plast Surg 1994;32:32.

8. Nahabedian MY, Momen B, Galdino G, et al. Breast reconstruction with the free TRAM or DIEP flap: patient selection, choice of flap, and outcome. Plast Reconstr Surg 2002;110:466–75.

9. Lipa J. Breast reconstruction with free flaps from the abdominal donor site – TRAM, DIEAP, and SIEA flaps. Clin Plast Surg 2007;34:105–21.

10. Grotting JC. The free abdominoplasty flap for immediate breast reconstruction. Ann Plast Surg 1991;27:351–4.

11. Granzow JW, Levine JL, Chiu ES, et al. Breast reconstruction with the deep inferior epigastric perforator flap: history and an update on current technique. J Plast Reconstr Aesthet Surg 2006;59:571–9.

12. De Frene B, Van Landuyt K, Hamdi M, et al. Free DIEAP and SGAP flap breast reconstruction after abdominal/gluteal liposuction. J Plast Reconstr Aesthet Surg 2006;59:1031–6.

13. Rogers N, Allen R. Radiation effects on breast reconstruction with the deep inferior epigastric perforator flap. Plast Reconstr Surg 2002;109:1919–24.

14. Blondeel PN. Deep inferior epigastric artery perforator flap. In: Blondeel PN, Morris SF, Hallock GG, et al, editors. In: Perforator flaps. Anatomy, techniques & clinical applications, vol. 1. St Louis (MO): Quality Medical Publishers, Inc.; 2006. p. 385–403.

15. Hamdi M, Rebecca A. The deep inferior epigastric artery perforator flap (DIEAP) in breast reconstruction. Semin Plast Surg 2006;20:95–102.

16. Blondeel PN. One hundred free DIEP flap breast reconstructions: a personal experience. Br J Plast Surg 1999;52:104–11.

17. Kroll SS. Fat necrosis in free transverse rectus abdominis myocutaneous and deep inferior epigastric perforator flaps. Plast Reconstr Surg 2000; 106:576–83.

18. Agarwal JP, Gottlieb LJ. Double pedicle deep inferior epigastric perforator/muscle-sparing TRAM flaps for unilateral breast reconstruction. Ann Plast Surg 2007;58:359–63.

19. Tseng CY, Lang PO, Cipriani NA. Pedicle preservation technique for arterial and venous turbocharging of free DIEP and muscle-sparing TRAM flaps. Plast Reconstr Surg 2007;120:851–4.

20. Gill P, Hunt J, Guerra A, et al. A 10-year retrospective review of 758 DIEP flaps for breast reconstruction. Plast Reconstr Surg 2004;113:1153–60.

21. Nahabedian MY, Tsangaris T, Momen B. Breast reconstruction with the DIEP flap or the muscle-sparing (MS-2) free TRAM flap: is there a difference? Plast Reconstr Surg 2005;115:436–44.

22. Chevray PM. Breast reconstruction with superficial inferior epigastric artery flaps: a prospective comparison with TRAM and DIEP flaps. Plast Reconstr Surg 2004;114:1077–83.

23. Spiegel AJ, Khan FN. An intraoperative algorithm for use of the SIEA flap for breast reconstruction. Plast Reconstr Surg 2007;120:1450–9.

24. Granzow JW, Levine JL, Chiu ES, et al. Breast reconstruction using perforator flaps. J Surg Oncol 2006; 94:441–54.

25. Holm C, Mayr M, Hofter E, et al. The versatility of the SIEA flap: a clinical assessment of the vascular territory of the superficial epigastric inferior artery. J Plast Reconstr Aesthet Surg 2007;60:946–51.

26. Guerra AB, Metzinger SE, Bidros RS. Breast reconstruction with gluteal artery perforator (GAP) flaps. A critical analysis of 142 cases. Ann Plast Surg 2004;52:118–25.

27. Shaw WW. Superior gluteal free flap breast reconstruction. Clin Plast Surg 1998;25:267–74.

28. Allen RJ, Tucker C. Superior gluteal artery perforator free flap for breast reconstruction. Plast Reconstr Surg 1995;95:1207–12.

29. Allen RJ, Levine JL, Granzow JW. The in-the-crease inferior gluteal artery perforator flap for breast reconstruction. Plast Reconstr Surg 2006;188:333–9.

30. Le-Quang C. Secondary microsurgical reconstruction of the breast and free inferior gluteal flap. Ann Chir Plast Esthet 1992;37:723.

31. Paletta CE, Bostwick J, Nahai F. The inferior gluteal free flap in breast reconstruction. Plast Reconstr Surg 1989;84:875.

32. Angrigiani C, Grilli D, Siebert J. Latissimus dorsi musculocutaneous flap without muscle. Plast Reconstr Surg 1995;96:1608–14.

33. Kerrigan CL, Daniel RK. The intercostal flap: an anatomical and hemodynamic approach. Ann Plast Surg 1979;2:411–21.

34. Hamdi M, de Frene B. Pedicled perforator flaps in breast reconstruction. Semin Plast Surg 2006; 20(2):73–8.

35. Heitmann C, Guerra A, Metzinger SW, et al. The thoracodorsal artery perforator flap: anatomic basis and clinical application. Ann Plast Surg 2003;51:23–9.

36. Hamdi M, Van Landuyt K, Hijjawi JB, et al. Surgical technique in pedicled thoracodorsal artery

perforator flaps: a clinical experience with 99 patients. Plast Reconstr Surg 2008;121:1632–41.

37. Hamdi M, Van Landuyt K, de Frene B, et al. The versatility of the intercostal artery perforator (ICAP) flap. J Plast Reconstr Aesthet Surg 2006;59:644–52.

38. Kwei S, Borud LJ, Lee BT. Mastopexy with autologous augmentation after massive weight loss: the intercostal artery perforator (ICAP) flap. Ann Plast Surg 2006;57:361–5.

39. Hamdi M, Van Landuyt K, Blondeel P, et al. Autologous breast augmentation with the lateral intercostal artery perforator flap in massive weight loss patients. J Plast Reconstr Aesthet Surg 2009;62:65–70.

40. Badran HA, El-Helaly MS, Safe I. The lateral intercostal neurovascular free flap. Plast Reconstr Surg 1984;73:17–26.

41. Hamdi M, Spano A, Van Landuyt K, et al. The lateral intercostal artery perforators: anatomical study and clinical application in breast surgery. Plast Reconstr Surg 2008;121:389–96.

42. Masia J, Clavero JA, Larranaga JR, et al. Multidetector-row computed tomography in the planning of abdominal perforator flaps. J Plast Reconstr Aesthet Surg 2006;59:594–9.

43. Karanas YL, Antony A, Rubin G, et al. Preoperative CT angiography for free fibula transfer. Microsurgery 2005;24:125–7.

44. Rozen WM, Phillips TJ, Ashton MW, et al. Preoperative imaging for DIEA perforator flaps: a comparative study of computed tomographic angiography and Doppler ultrasound. Plast Reconstr Surg 2008;121: 9–16.

45. Rozen WM, Ashton MW, Grinsell D, et al. Establishing the case for CT angiography in the preoperative imaging of abdominal wall perforators. Microsurgery 2008;28:306–13.

46. Scheinfeld NS, Cowper SE. Nephrogenic fibrosing dermopathy. Available at: http://www.emedicine. corn/derm/topic934.htm; Accessed July 2, 2010.

47. Greenspun D, Vasile J, Levine JL, et al. Anatomic imaging of abdominal perforator flaps without ionizing radiation: seeing is believing with magnetic resonance imaging angiography. J Reconstr Microsurg 2010;26(1):37–44.

48. Vasile J, Newman T, Rusch DG, et al. Anatomic imaging of gluteal perforator flaps without ionizing radiation: seeing is believing with magnetic resonance angiography. J Reconstr Microsurg 2010; 26(1):45–57.

49. Neil-Dwyer JG, Ludman CN, Schaverien M, et al. Magnetic resonance angiography in preoperative planning of deep inferior epigastric artery perforator flaps. J Plast Reconstr Aesthet Surg 2009;62(12): 1661–5.

Pedicled Perforator Flaps in the Trunk

Moustapha Hamdi, MD, PhD, FCCP*,
Filip B.J.L. Stillaert, MD, FCCP

KEYWORDS

- Trunk defects • Musculocutaneous perforators
- Thoracodorsal artery • Latissimus dorsi

Trunk defects can be approached through a multitude of regional flaps that can be harvested from the shoulder girdle, epigastric axis, paraspinal region, or pelvic girdle. The aim of the reconstruction is to provide adequate and tension-free restoration of tissue integrity with minimal functional morbidity, water- and air-tight closure of cavities, and coverage of exposed vital structures.[1,2] The reconstructive modus operandi is directed by the location, size, and cause of the defect as well as the availability of healthy, adjacent autogenous graft tissue.[3] Potential donor sites should be estimated for their tissue quality and anticipated donor site morbidity in proportion to the surgical indication and general condition of the patient. The patency of the source vessels of likely flaps should be acknowledged for impairment by previous surgery. However, the larger the defect the greater the need to include several pedicled flaps or consider free microsurgical tissue transfer. The prototypical pedicled flap has a constant, reliable anatomy. However, it should have a versatile configuration that is adequate for coverage and resistant to infection. Also, the surgical technique should be uncomplicated.

CHOICE OF FLAPS
Muscle Flaps

In the late nineteenth century, Tansini used a latissimus dorsi (LD) muscle flap for primary breast and chest wall reconstruction, and the reliable pedicled LD flap with its modifications has become a time-honored constituent of the reconstructive armamentarium.[4] Although several investigators have largely described the use of muscle flaps to manage tissue defects of the trunk,[5–7] some more-complicated defects in specific areas on the trunk can be difficult to reach with pedicled muscle or myocutaneous flaps. These regions are (1) the posterolateral iliac crest region, especially when associated with a volume of iliac bone loss, (2) the epigastric axis and upper quadrants, which can require great effort to reconstruct with pedicle flaps because the rib cage makes mobilization of local flaps difficult (omentum is available if soft tissue coverage is needed in those areas as in the rectus abdominis muscle), (3) the lower lumbar and upper sacral regions can be difficult to approach because of distal reach and potential interference with muscles that are important for ambulation, and (4) the upper back and lower-cervical region may be problematic to reach with regional flaps, especially for larger defects, and the tissue bulk provided by the trapezius muscle or rhomboid muscles may be limited for such defects.

Axial Pattern Flaps

The repertoire of skin flaps used to be limited to random flaps, which were raised without regard to any known blood supply other than the subdermal plexus. Those flaps were restricted to rigid length-to-width ratios to ensure viability. After McGregor and Morgan introduced the concept of axial flaps, Ger and Duboys[7] soon popularized the use of muscle as a carrier of overlying skin to create larger myocutaneous flaps. Knowledge of the intrinsic blood supply has been recognized

Department of Plastic and Reconstructive Surgery, University Hospital Gent, De Pintelaan 185, Gent 9000, Belgium
* Corresponding author.
E-mail address: moustapha.hamdi@ugent.be

Clin Plastic Surg 37 (2010) 655–665
doi:10.1016/j.cps.2010.06.004

as the most important determinant for ensuring success in elevating cutaneous flaps, and many of the previously described myocutaneous flaps can be harvested as skin flaps based on their perforators.

Perforator Flaps

Progress in reconstructive surgery has refined standard procedures, and the introduction of perforator flap surgery has extended the arsenal of reliable and safe surgical preferences to achieve primary closure of trunk defects. The concept of the freestyle perforator flap surgery offers even greater flexibility to choose the donor site, because flap selection is based on the quality and volume of soft tissue required at the recipient site (**Fig. 1**).[8] After evaluating the defect, an appropriate area adjacent to the injury site is selected and Doppler investigation and mapping are performed followed by custom-made flap design.

REGIONAL BLOOD SUPPLY

The vascular anatomy of the trunk is represented by the following: the chest, abdomen, upper back, and lumbar regions. The chest region extends from the clavicles to the costal margins and laterally up to the midaxillary line. The abdominal region extends from the costal margin to the iliac crest, the inguinal ligament, and the pubis anteriorly and is delineated from the upper back and lumbar regions by the midaxillary line. The upper back region extends superiorly to a line joining the C7 spinous process with the acromial angle and inferiorly to the lower margin of the 12th rib. The lumbar region extends from this inferior boundary of the upper back region to a line joining the 2 posterior superior iliac spines and along the iliac crest. The arterial blood supply of the trunk arises from 3 primary arterial systems: the subclavian/axillary axis, the descending aorta, and the external iliac arteries. Superiorly, branches from the subclavian/axillary axis supply the chest, axilla, and part of the upper back. Posteriorly, the descending thoracic and abdominal aorta give off the segmental posterior intercostal, subcostal, and lumbar arteries. Inferiorly, perforators from the epigastric and circumflex iliac branches supply the lower abdomen. Perforators of the integument of the trunk originate from 17 source arteries (average of 122 ± perforators)[9] with most being musculocutaneous, originating from the primary blood supply of the broad superficial muscles in this region. Several septocutaneous perforators arise from the perimeter of these muscles and from near the joint creases of the extremities

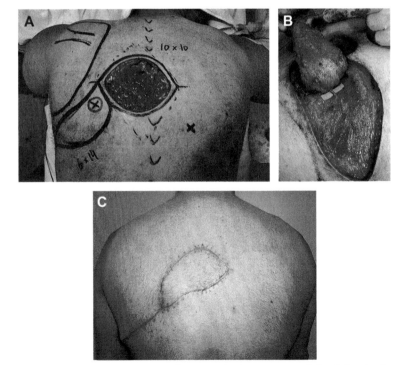

Fig. 1. (*A*) Excision of a basocellular carcinoma at the upper back. Coverage of the defect is planned with a free-style intercostal artery perforator flap. The flap is rotated 180° into the defect. (*B*) The perforator is completely isolated to achieve maximum mobilization of the flap. (*C*) Two months postoperation.

where the skin is tethered to underlying connective tissue. The large septocutaneous perforators are easily distinguished in angiograms of the integument because they frequently have a larger diameter and travel greater distances, thus supplying large vascular territories. The ratio of musculocutaneous to septocutaneous perforators is 4:1. The average diameter and area supplied by a single perforator from the trunk region are approximately $0.7 + 0.2$ mm and 40 ± 15 cm^2, respectively.[9]

Both unidirectional Doppler flowmetry and color duplex scanning have proved to be useful tools in evaluating the vascular anatomy preoperatively, improving surgical planning, and reducing operating time.[10] Multidetector computed tomography (CT)-based imaging has provided detailed information on the quality, course, and localization in the form of 3-dimensional images of the perforators. The high sensitivity and specificity of the technique make it possible to select the preferred perforator preoperatively, effectively improving surgical strategy and reducing valuable operating time and postoperative complications.[11]

REGIONAL OVERVIEW
Chest

Regional muscle flaps to address anteriorly located trunk defects are the turnover pectoralis major (PM) muscle flap, the advanced PM muscle flap, the LD muscle flap, the omentum flap, and the rectus abdominis muscle flap. Lateral chest wall defects can be approached using the PM muscle flap, the LD flap, the serratus anterior flap, the omentum flap, and the superiorly based rectus abdominis flap, whereas the pelvic girdle regional flaps for torso reconstruction are the external oblique muscle flap, groin flap, inferiorly based rectus abdominis muscle flap, rectus femoris muscle flap, tensor fascia lata flap, and gracilis muscle flap.

Musculocutaneous perforators of the internal thoracic artery, thoracoacromial artery, and lateral rami of the posterior intercostal arteries and septocutaneous perforators from the lateral thoracic artery and thyrocervical trunk supply the skin envelope of the chest. The superficial thoracic branch of the lateral thoracic artery and the large anterior intercostal perforators of the internal thoracic or mammary artery supply most of the integument of the lateral, medial, and intermediate regions of the anterior chest wall. Musculocutaneous perforators from the clavicular and deltoid arteries and variable septocutaneous vessels from the transverse cervical, suprascapular, and supraclavicular branches of the thyrocervical trunk supply the superior integument of the chest.

Perforators arising from the clavicular and deltoid branches of the thoracoacromial artery could be suitable for perforator flap harvest compared with perforators from the pectoral branch.[12]

Musculocutaneous perforators from the internal thoracic or mammary artery together with its anterior intercostal branches supply the greater part of the anterior chest wall. Of clinical concern are the second, third, and fourth intercostal musculocutaneous perforators. In their anatomic study, Geddes and colleagues[12] showed an average number of 5 ± 2 perforators greater than 0.5 mm in diameter, supplying an area of 183 ± 61 cm^2 or 8% of the integument of the trunk.

Internal mammary artery perforator flap

Bakamijan[13] based his deltopectoral flap medially over the internal mammary artery perforators (IMAPs). The territory of the IMAP flap, corresponding to that of the deltopectoral flap, extends along 3 angiosomes of the anterior chest and shoulder. The average size of the IMAP flap is 13×7 cm up to 20×13 cm.[14] The unique blood supply to the IMAP flap is derived from the perforators of the internal mammary vessels that pierce the intercostal muscles and PM muscle just lateral to the sternum. The orientation of the skin flap can be alternated because the perforator also sends branches obliquely inferiorly. Usually, the perforator in the second intercostal space is the largest.[14] Because there is a large variability in the diameter of the lower perforators, preoperative mapping with Doppler ultrasonography or angio-CT scan is advisable. The efficacy in harvesting this large cutaneous flap is because of the laterally directed course of the perforators with their generous distal collateralization. During flap elevation, the deep fascia should be preserved because its rich vascularization ensures survival of the lateral portion of the IMAP flap. The internal mammary artery gives rise to perforators through each intercostal space to supply the overlying skin and allows multiple flap freestyle configurations and flap designs. The IMAP flap can be deflected cranially or rotated to the opposite side and its arc of rotation can be improved if the perforator is dissected out until the mammary artery. This flap provides skin of comparable color and texture for anterior neck reconstructions.[15,16] The commonly used myocutaneous PM flap often provides a skin flap that is too thick, barely reaches the distal wound, and is often difficult to model. The second and third IMAPs support a large flap that covers the entire lateral cervical triangle up to the submandibular region. Direct closure of the donor site can often be achieved, but for larger areas, either preoperative skin expansion or skin grafting may be necessary.[17] When elevated on the lower perforators, the skin area of IMAP 4 covers the inframammary fold region. The use of the IMAP flap based on the fourth IMAP is suitable for patients in whom a breast reconstruction in combination with a reduction mammaplasty on the contralateral side is needed. Otherwise, discarded tissue during reduction mammaplasty is transposed from the submammary fold to the contralateral side. The resulting scar is well hidden and donor site morbidity optimized.[14]

Anterior intercostal artery perforator flap

The intercostal vessels form an arcade, which can be divided into 4 segments: vertebral, intercostal, intermuscular, and rectus segments. The anterior intercostal artery arises from the internal mammary artery (first through sixth intercostal spaces) or from its musculophrenic branch (seventh through ninth intercostal spaces). The 2 lowest intercostal spaces have only posterior arteries. The anterior intercostal vessels eventually communicate with the posterior intercostal vessels at the anteromedial one-third of the ribs. Perforators pierce the upper 5 or 6 intercostal spaces; those perforators of the second through fourth spaces are large in women and supply the breast. The perforator can be located with Doppler investigation within a 1- to 3-cm area lateral to the sternal border. The flap is designed around the perforator, usually longitudinally or obliquely, toward the shoulder. The flap is dissected from lateral to medial and distal to cranial directions. If a long pedicle is required, further dissection in the costal groove is necessary, which can be quite difficult because of adherent vessels. A sensate flap can be elevated by including the intercostal nerve. The flap can be used for sternal, breast, or thoracic defects as a transposition island flap. It can also be transferred as V-Y advancement flap for distal (epigastric) or lateral defects.

The thoracodorsal artery perforator flap

First described by Angrigiani and colleagues[18] in 1995, the thoracodorsal artery perforator (TDAP) flap has a lengthy, reliable, and sizeable pedicle that is constant. The thoracodorsal artery (TDA) is a terminal branch of the subscapular artery dividing into a transverse and descending branch. The vascular territory of the TDAP flap essentially lies on top of the LD muscle. The musculocutaneous perforators normally originate from the descending branch, which follows the lateral border of the muscle inferiorly. The main perforator does not need to be centered to reliably perfuse the pedicled perforator flap because it has been proved that the skin island in the classical myocutaneous LD flap can extend beyond the border of the muscle and skin flaps measuring up to 14 × 25 cm have been used without complications.[19] Furthermore, the skin island can be oriented in different directions depending on the reconstructive requirements and anticipated direction of the scar. The flap is particularly useful for resurfacing large defects of the trunk because of its long vascular pedicle and minimal donor site morbidity (**Fig. 2**).[20,21] The trunk's large skin territory is attributed to the fact that the main perforators are widely prevalent in the region, and this arrangement creates larger angiosomes increasing the vascular territory of each perforator.[22] With the patient in a lateral decubitus position, the anterior border of the LD muscle is palpated and marked. The anterior border of the TDAP flap should be set out in front of the LD muscle border at the level of the vascular hilus, which is about 8 cm below the axillary crease. This design includes potential cutaneous branches of the TDA. The flap is outlined as a vertical ellipse over the LD muscle. Most perforators tend to exit the muscle during the course of the descending branch of the TDA, which can lead to false-positive results using Doppler investigation. The initial incision is made at the anteroinferior border of the flap to identify the anterior border of the LD muscle and if necessary, to reposition this border accordingly. If more than 1 perforator is found, the required pedicle length (and location of the recipient site) determines which vessel is chosen. Some of the more distal perforators can originate from the intercostal vessels. To determine whether this is the case, the anterior border of the LD muscle should be freed and the underside inspected.

The lateral intercostal artery perforator flap

The lateral intercostal neurovascular pedicle flap was first described as a musculocutaneous flap[23] and later as a perforator flap.[24] The intercostal neurovascular segment of the arcade formed by the intercostal vessels is the longest (12 cm) and it gives rise to between 5 and 7 musculocutaneous perforators. A variable number of intercostal perforators can be used clinically in an area between the LD and PM muscles.[25] A dominant perforator can be identified, especially in the fourth to eighth intercostal spaces, with a higher concentration in the sixth and seventh intercostal spaces. These dominant perforators are located on an average of 3.5 cm from the anterior border of the LD muscle.[25] The lateral intercostal artery perforator (LICAP)

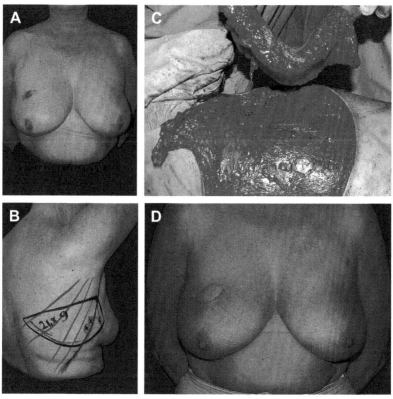

Fig. 2. (*A*) Preoperative view before quadrantectomy (upper lateral) for mammary gland tumor. (*B*) Design of a TDAP on the LD muscle. Three perforators have been identified using Doppler ultrasonography. (*C*) Intraoperative view on the perforator on which the flap is based. (*D*) Postoperative view with restoration of the contour of the mammary gland.

flap is a good alternative to the TDAP flap in reconstructing lateral quadrant defects of the breast.[25,26] The lateral branches of the posterior intercostal arteries supply musculocutaneous perforators to the lateral lumbar and abdominal region from the 8th through 11th arteries and subcostal segmental origins. The expansive network of cutaneous anastomoses, the reliability of the deep pedicle, and the abundance of tissue in this loose-skinned region of the abdomen give these vessels a great deal of potential for perforator flap harvest with great versatility. The intercostal vessels can be dissected within the intercostal groove to obtain a longer pedicle, but this procedure can be tedious and time consuming. As an alternative, a longer pedicle can be obtained if the flap is based on the connection between the intercostal and the serratus anterior vessels. A serratus anterior artery perforator flap has 6 to 9 cm of pedicle length, giving it a useful arc of rotation well into the region of the areola.[25] Hamdi and colleagues[25] showed in their cadaver study that this connection is present in only 21% of cases.

Abdomen

The superior, deep inferior, and superficial epigastric arteries (SEA, DIEA, and SIEA); lateral intercostal perforators; and deep and superficial circumflex iliac arteries (DCIA and SCIA) supply the abdominal region.

The superior epigastric artery perforator flap

The SEA continues inferiorly along the same line as the internal thoracic artery. The SEA has an average number of 5 ± 1 perforators supplying the superior abdominal region and emerging in most cases in a zone immediately below the costal margin, up to the first tendinous insertion of the rectus abdominis muscle (**Fig. 3**). The superficial branch of the SEA, which pierces the rectus fascia directly under the xiphoid toward the skin, has the potential to provide the vascular basis for a perforator flap.[27] However, the pedicle length is short because it is hindered by the proximity of the artery to the sternum and ribs. Flaps based on the superficial branch are useful for the reconstruction of presternal defects. Manchot[28] originally described this branch as the superficial

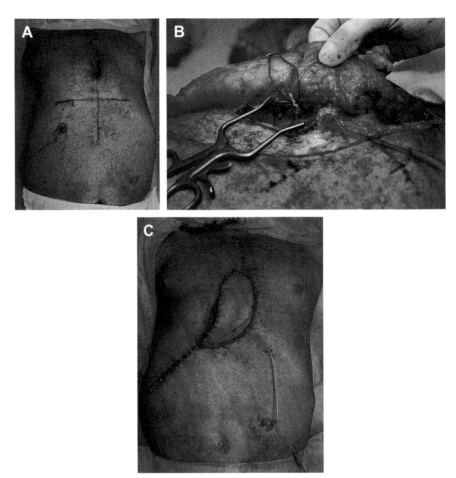

Fig. 3. (A) Preoperative marking of a superior epigastric artery perforator (SEAP) on which a SEAP flap is based to cover a sternal defect. (B) Intraoperative view of the perforator. (C) Immediate postoperative result. Coverage of the sternal defect was achieved through 180° rotation of the SEAP flap.

SEA. The main trunk of the SEA enters the rectus abdominis muscle on its deep surface, approximately 7 cm below the costal margin. Multidetector angio-CT scan can easily distinguish between perforators arising from the deep SEA and those arising from the intercostals or even those from the costomarginal artery, which branches out of the lateral division of the deep SEA and its anastomosis with the eighth posterior intercostal artery.[27]

Deep inferior epigastric artery perforator flap

The deep inferior epigastric artery perforator (DIEAP) flap is versatile to reconstruct defects in the lower abdominal and inguinofemoral regions. The flap has a long and reliable pedicle and provides pliable and healthy tissue bulk. The DIEAP flap is a versatile approach also to reconstruct defects in the groin region and the proximal upper leg region can be harvested as well as an ipsilateral

or contralateral flap. Coverage with healthy tissue in the groin is preferable to protect the underlying neurovascular bundles in an area of high mobility (**Figs. 4** and **5**).

Upper Back

Obtaining stable tissue coverage of posterior cervicothoracic defects can be challenging, because the back is a region of high tensile and traction forces. In this area, the selection of flaps for coverage depends on a thorough understanding of the anatomy, the assessment of the arc of rotation, and the location of the defect as well as its size and extension (see **Fig. 1**).[29] The back provides thin pliable tissue with minimal bulk. Possible pedicled muscle or myocutaneous flaps to be used for back reconstruction are the LD flap, the distally based turndown LD flap, the trapezius flap, and the rhomboid major flap. Five

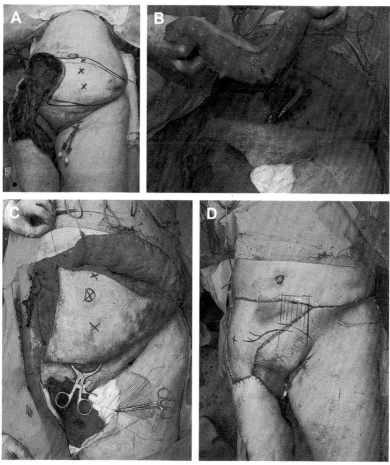

Fig. 4. A 54-year-old patient is shown after several aggressive debridement procedures to control a necrotizing fasciitis (*A*). The perforators on the abdomen were located using Doppler ultrasonography, and the best perforator was selected for the prelevation of a DIEAP flap (*B, C*). A pedicled contralateral DIEAP flap could easily cover the resultant defect and the neurovascular structures (*D*).

major source vessels provide the musculocutaneous perforators supplying the upper back region: the thyrocervical trunk with the transverse and deep cervical arteries superiorly, the subscapular axis branches laterally, and the posterior intercostal arteries medially. The upper back region has an average of 24 perforators, each supplying a skin territory of approximately 40 cm². Perforator flaps reported in this area are the TDAP flap, the DICAP flap, the septocutaneous circumflex scapular artery (CSA) perforator flap, the dorsal scapular artery perforator (DSAP) flap (infra), and the subcostal artery perforator (SCAP) flap.

The DSAP flap

The dorsal scapular artery originates from the subclavian artery as an independent branch or from the trunk of the transverse cervical artery and supplies the medial area of the lower back.[30] Angrigiani and colleagues[31] have found that a dorsal scapular island (perforator) flap can be

raised on this vessel with a pedicle of up to 16 cm. The DSAP flap transfers skin and subcutaneous tissue from the back to the anterior neck, face, and thoracic wall with minimal morbidity, sparing the trapezius muscle completely. The flap is based on the cutaneous perforator of the dorsal scapular artery and vein. This perforator is consistently present[31] and courses under the trapezius muscle and under the omohyoid and levator scapulae muscles on top of the rib cage.[29] The perforator's superficial branch pierces the rhomboideus at the level of the medial angle of the scapula and appears under the deep surface of the trapezius muscle. The flap is based on the superficial branch. After giving off this superficial branch, the main trunk of the dorsal scapular artery becomes the deep branch of the dorsal scapular artery. The flap has a long pedicle (15–16 cm) and can be tunneled under the main portion of the trapezius, levator scapulae, and omohyoideus muscles, to reach the anterior thoracic wall,

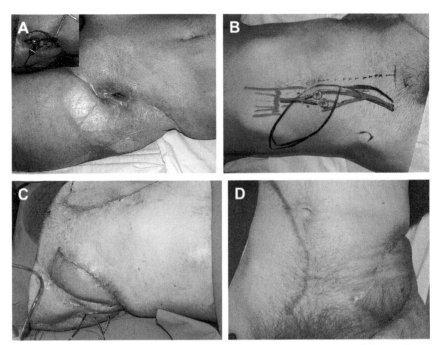

Fig. 5. A 33-year-old man who underwent a radical resection for a pelvic sarcoma with hip replacement by a cemented prosthesis. Radiotherapy was given postoperatively, and wounds were complicated with chronic infection and fistula. The wound was debrided and a pedicled DIEAP/rectus abdominis muscle chimera flap was transferred. The rectus segment was wrapped around the prosthesis, and the skin paddle of the DIEAP flap was used to cover the defect. (*A*) Preoperative view shows the chronic fistula and after debridement (upper left corner). (*B*) The DIEAP/rectus abdominis muscle chimera flap was designed on the contralateral side. (*C*) The flap was transferred under the skin tunnel to cover the wound. (*D*) Complete wound healing was obtained with a follow-up of 6 months postoperatively.

cheek, and neck. The perforator of the dorsal scapular artery is usually located at the intersection of a line drawn 6 to 8 cm inferior to the spine of the scapula with a vertical line drawn 8 to 9 cm lateral to the midline of the back. The flap can be oriented in any direction and flaps as large as 20 × 20 cm can be safely harvested from this perforator.

The circumflex scapular artery perforator flap
The CSA originates from the subscapular artery along the lateral border of the scapula and gives rise to a large cutaneous perforator to the skin in the triangular space. This cutaneous perforator divides into 2 distinctive rami at the level of the deep fascia: the transverse (horizontal) branch (scapular cutaneous artery) and descending (vertical) branch (parascapular cutaneous artery). The scapular and parascapular flaps are based on the direct cutaneous branches of the CSA.

The dorsal intercostal artery perforator flap
Nine pairs of posterior intercostal arteries originate from the posterolateral aspect of the thoracic aorta. Nutrient musculocutaneous branches from

the 7th through the 11th intercostal and subcostal arteries emerge from the costal groove to supply the integument overlying the muscle. The anatomy and course of the intercostal vessels have been studied thoroughly in the anatomic work by Kerrigan and Daniel.[23] Perforators arising from the dorsal branches of the posterior intercostal arteries can supply pedicled flaps for local reconstruction in the paraspinal region (see **Fig. 5**). Depending on their perforator location, the intercostal artery perforator flaps are classified as follows

- DICAP: based on the perforators that arise from the vertebral segment. These flaps can be designed near the midline of the back.
- LICAP: based on the perforators that arise from the costal segment.
- AICAP: based on the perforators that arise from the muscular or rectal segments.

The posterior intercostal arteries form the largest angiosome in the torso by their many perforators.[32] Among these intercostal artery perforators, there consistently exist fairly large perforators along the dorsal midline. Such large perforators are large enough to supply island flaps, which can be called DICAP flaps.[33] The upper DICAP flaps (fourth, fifth, and sixth DICAPs) can safely be extended as far as the midaxillary line or the anterior border of LD, because they capture a large vascular territory of the scapular circumflex artery or the thoracodorsal artery by choke anastomoses.[33] The lower 10th and 11th DICAPs descend parallel to the costal angle and form choke anastomoses with the cutaneous branches of the lumbar arteries or musculocutaneous perforators of the LD, extending their vascular territories reachable to the iliac crest as the caudal limitation. The lower DICAPs thus show more vertical axiality than the upper perforators. Less dominant are the seventh, eighth, and ninth intercostal artery perforators. These perforators tend to send the distal segmental muscular branches to the LD rather than sending the direct cutaneous perforators. Doppler probe auscultation within 5 cm lateral to the spinous processes of the vertebrae can detect the dorsal LICAPs (see **Fig. 5**). The perimeter of the DICAP flap is marked from the dorsal midline along the axes of the ribs. The distal end of the DICAP flap must be set within the lateral margin of the LD muscle for upper DICAP flaps or the iliac crest for lower DICAP flaps. The dissection of the DICAP flap can easily be performed creating a fasciocutaneous flap. The deep fascia is dispensable for the vascularity of the flap but including it in the flap makes the dissection easier and more secure. The DICAP flap can easily be rotated with the versatile swing arc on the perforator as a pedicle of the island flap. Extra length can be gained by intramuscular dissection of the DICAP to meet the distance to the recipient site. The donor site can be closed primarily up to a width of 8 cm.

Lumbar-Subcostal Region

Coverage of tissue defects in the lumbosacral region is a difficult task. In this area, the skin is very tight and direct closure by simple undermining is only feasible for small defects because of the high tensile and traction forces in this area.

SCAP flap
The SCAP flap has a long pedicle allowing a large arc of rotation, and midline defects in the lower back can be covered without any tension.[31] The vascular basis for this fasciocutaneous flap is the subcostal artery, which corresponds to the 12th thoracic segment. The artery's lateral cutaneous branch descends caudally from the 12th rib and emerges through the fascia of the external oblique muscle at the lateral border of the LD muscle up to

3 cm below the 12th rib. The lateral cutaneous branch supplies the skin of the flank between the lower rib and the anterior superior iliac spine (ASIS).[32] The subcostal artery is absent in 5% of cases and is usually replaced by a branch from the 11th intercostal artery.[33]

The lumbar artery perforator flap
Four lumbar arteries originate from the descending abdominal aorta as paired segmental branches, opposite the bodies of the upper 4 lumbar vertebral bodies and in the vicinity of the lateral border of the erector spinae. Medial and lateral branches are sent from these vessels as septocutaneous perforators between the abdominal muscles and the erector spinae muscles. The lateral branches are large and supply the integument lateral to the posterior midline. The lumbar artery perforator–based island flap has advantages because it is a fasciocutaneous flap based on a single artery. The flap does not sacrifice any muscle, has a large rotational arc, and its donor site can be closed primarily. The injection study by Kato and colleagues[34] showed that the skin territory of the second lumbar artery alone was from the posterior midline to the lateral border of the rectus sheath and was at least 10 cm above the ASIS. When a large flap is needed, the flap may be designed so that the axis of the flap runs obliquely from the midline down to the ASIS, because the lumbar arteries anastomose with each other and form a vascular network. The high mobility of this flap enables it to be used for the lower back as well as the thoracic spinal region and posterior costal region reconstruction.

SUMMARY

Large defects of the integument of the trunk can be approached through elevation of perforator flaps with great reliability. The choice of a certain perforator flap basically depends on the location and size of the defect while considering the effect of the donor site morbidity on functional and aesthetic outcomes. Evaluation of the reconstructive options must include consideration of previously placed surgical scars, the anatomic location of the defect, analysis of the defect itself (requiring bulk structural support or covering vital structures), and unavailability of regional flaps, the use of which may be precluded by tumor ablation or irradiation. Under these circumstances, some investigators have advocated microvascular reconstruction. However, with the concept of perforator flaps, some innovative flap designs and techniques have been developed to address most of the torso defects. Pedicled perforator flaps offer reliable and satisfactory results of reconstruction at different anatomic territories of the torso.

REFERENCES

1. Tukiainen E, Popov P, Asko-Seljavaara S. Microvascular reconstruction of full-thickness oncological chest wall defects. Ann Surg 2003;238(6): 794–802.
2. Netscher DT, Valkov PL. Reconstruction of oncologic torso defects: emphasis on microvascular reconstruction. Semin Surg Oncol 2000;19(3):255–63.
3. Losken A, Thourani VH, Carlson GW, et al. A reconstructive algorithm for plastic surgery following extensive chest wall resection. Br J Plast Surg 2004;57(4):295–302.
4. Saint-Cyr M, Nagarkar P, Schaverien M, et al. The pedicled descending branch muscle-sparing latissimus dorsi flap for breast reconstruction. Plast Reconstr Surg 2009;123(1):13–24.
5. Kanavel AB. Plastic procedures for the obliteration of cavities with non-collapsible walls. Surg Gynecol Obstet 1921;32:453–9.
6. Wangensteen OH. Repair of recurrent and difficult hernias and other large defects of the abdominal wall employing the iliac tibial tract of fascia lata as a pedicled flap. Surg Gynecol Obstet 1934;59: 766–80.
7. Ger R, Duboys E. The prevention and repair of large abdominal-wall defects by muscle transposition: a preliminary communication. Plast Reconstr Surg 1983;72(2):170–8.
8. Bravo GB, Schwarze HP. Free-style local perforator flaps: concept and classification system. J Plast Reconstr Aesthet Surg 2009;62(5):602–8.
9. Geddes CR, Tang M, Yang D, et al. Anatomy of the integument of the trunk. In: Blondeel PN, Morris SF, Hallock GG, et al, editors. Perforator flaps, anatomy, technique & clinical applications. Missouri: Quality Medical Publishing; 2006. p. 360–84.
10. Hallock GG. Doppler sonography and color duplex imaging for planning a perforator flap. Clin Plast Surg 2003;30(3):347–57.
11. Masia J, Clavero JA, Larranaga JR, et al. Multidetector-row computed tomography in the planning of abdominal perforator flaps. J Plast Reconstr Aesthet Surg 2006;59(6):594–9.
12. Geddes CR, Tang M, Yang D, et al. An assessment of the anatomical basis of the thoracoacromial artery perforator flap. Can J Plast Surg 2003;11:23–7.
13. Bakamijan VY. A two-stage method for pharyngooesophageal reconstruction with a primary pectoral skin flap. Plast Reconstr Surg 1965;36:173–84.
14. Schmidt M, Aszmann OC, Beck H, et al. The anatomic basis of the internal mammary artery perforator flap: a cadaver study. J Plast Reconstr Aesthet Surg 2010;63:191–6.
15. Neligan PC, Gullane PJ, Vesely M, et al. The internal mammary artery perforator flap: new variation on an old theme. Plast Reconstr Surg 2007; 119(3):891–3.
16. Yu P, Roblin P, Chevray P. Internal mammary artery perforator (IMAP) flap for tracheostoma reconstruction. Head Neck 2006;28(8):723–9.
17. Saint-Cyr M, Schaverien M, Rohrich RJ. Preexpanded second intercostal space internal mammary artery pedicle perforator flap: case report and anatomical study. Plast Reconstr Surg 2009;123(6): 1659–64.
18. Angrigiani C, Grilli D, Siebert J. Latissimus dorsi musculocutaneous flap without muscle. Plast Reconstr Surg 1995;96(7):1608–14.
19. Van Landuyt K, Hamdi M. Thoracodorsal artery perforator flap. In: Blondeel PN, Morris SF, Hallock GG, et al, editors. Perforator flaps, anatomy, technique & clinical applications. Missouri: Quality Medical Publishing; 2006. p. 442–59.
20. Hamdi M, Van Landuyt K, Hijawi JB, et al. Surgical technique in pedicled thoracodorsal artery perforator flaps: a clinical experience with 99 patients. Plast Reconstr Surg 2008;121(5):1632–41.
21. Hamdi M, Decorte T, Demuynck M, et al. Shoulder function after harvesting a thoracodorsal artery perforator flap. Plast Reconstr Surg 2008;122(4): 1111–7.
22. Heitmann C, Guerra A, Metzinger SW, et al. The thoracodorsal artery perforator flap: anatomical basis and clinical applications. Ann Plast Surg 2003; 51(1):23–9.
23. Kerrigan CL, Daniel RK. The intercostal flap: an anatomical and hemodynamic approach. Ann Plast Surg 1979;2(5):411–21.
24. Badran HA, El-Helaly MS, Safe I. The lateral intercostal neurovascular free flap. Plast Reconstr Surg 1984;73(1):17–26.
25. Hamdi M, Spano A, Van Landuyt K, et al. The lateral intercostal artery perforators: anatomical study and clinical application in breast surgery. Plast Reconstr Surg 2008;121(2):389–96.
26. Hamdi M, Van Landuyt K, de Frene B, et al. The versatility of the intercostal artery perforator (ICAP) flaps. J Plast Reconstr Aesthet Surg 2006;59(6): 644–52.
27. Hamdi M, Van Landuyt K, Ulens S, et al. Clinical applications of the superior epigastric artery perforator (SEAP) flap: anatomical studies and preoperative perforator mapping with multidetector CT. J Plast Reconstr Aesthet Surg 2009;62(9):1127–34.
28. Manchot K. Die Hautarterien des Meslichen Korpers. Liepzig (Germany): FCW Vogel; 1889.
29. Stillaert FB, Van Landuyt K. Stable coverage of a cervico-thoracic defect with an extended lower

trapezius myocutaneous flap. J Plast Reconstr Aesthet Surg 2009;62(5):e101–2.

30. Tan KC, Tan BK. Extended lower trapezius island myocutaneous flap: a fasciomyocutaneous flap based on the dorsal scapular artery. Plast Reconstr Surg 2000;105(5):1758–63.

31. Angrigiani C, Grilli D, Karanas YL, et al. The dorsal scapular island flap: an alternative for head, neck, and chest reconstruction. Plast Reconstr Surg 2003;111(1):67–78.

32. Taylor GI, Minabe T. The angiosomes of the mammals and other vertebrates. Plast Reconstr Surg 1992;89(2):181–215.

33. Minabe T, Harii K. Dorsal intercostal artery perforator flap: anatomical study and clinical applications. Plast Reconstr Surg 2007;120(3):681–9.

34. Kato H, Hasegawa M, Takada T, et al. The lumbar artery perforator based island flap: anatomical study and case reports. Br J Plast Surg 1999; 52(7):541 6.

Perforator Flaps in the Upper Extremity

Michael Sauerbier, MD, PhD[a],*, Frank Unglaub, MD[b]

KEYWORDS

- Perforator flaps • Upper extremity • Vascular anatomy
- Defect coverage • Intrinsic flaps

Perforator flaps are frequently used for defect coverage for the whole body.[1] There are strong indications for the use of perforator flaps in the upper extremity.[2] This article demonstrates the possibilities for defect coverage with perforator flaps as well as their anatomic and technical considerations.

The following perforator flaps are described: lateral arm perforator, posterior interosseous artery perforator, ulnar artery perforator, radial artery perforator, radial artery fascial perforator, and intrinsic hand. General aspects of perforator flaps, including the anatomy at the upper limb are enumerated below.

- At the forearm, most of the blood supply comes from fasciocutaneous (direct) perforators that arise from the radial, ulnar, anterior interosseous, and posterior interosseous arteries. There are only few musculocutaneous (indirect) perforators.[3]
- Radial artery, ulnar artery, and anterior and posterior interosseous arteries supply the lower arm and the hand. In **Fig. 1** the individual areas are drawn in. **Fig. 2** shows important perforators of different forearm arteries.
- The palmar aspect of the hand is supplied predominantly by the ulnar artery through the superficial palmar arch. The dorsal part of the hand is supplied by the radial artery through the dorsal metacarpal arteries, which have communicating branches with the palmar arch. The digital arteries are arising from the arches in the hand and supply the fingers and thumb.
- Transversal anastomoses between perforators emerge from different main arteries, but mostly the longitudinal anastomoses realized between perforators emerge from the same principal artery are significant from the vascular point of view.[3,4]
- The distal third of the forearm has a rich supply of smaller caliber arterial perforators compared with the proximal two thirds of the forearm.[3] The proximal forearm, having larger perforators that branch to cover a larger surface area, is a source available for large flaps based on a single perforator. In the distal forearm, the perforators are of smaller caliber and would, therefore, tend to support smaller flaps.[5]
- Depending on their composition, the flaps can be cutaneous, subcutaneous, fasciosubcutaneous, and fascial.
- Perforator vessels supply not only the skin, but also the anatomic sector spanning between the skin and bone; these sectors are well known as angiotomes[6] or angiosomes[7] and represent the anatomical base of composite flaps in the forearm.
- Perforator flaps can be used in three major ways:
1. Pedicled flaps
2. Transposition flaps
3. Free flaps.

[a] Department for Plastic, Hand and Reconstructive Surgery, Main-Taunus Hospitals GmbH, Academic Hospital University of Frankfurt, Kronberger Strasse 36, 65812 Bad Soden am Taunus, Germany
[b] Department for Plastic and Hand Surgery, University Erlangen, Krankenhausstrasse 12, 91054 Erlangen, Germany
* Corresponding author.
E-mail address: msauerbier@kliniken-mtk.de

Clin Plastic Surg 37 (2010) 667–676
doi:10.1016/j.cps.2010.06.010

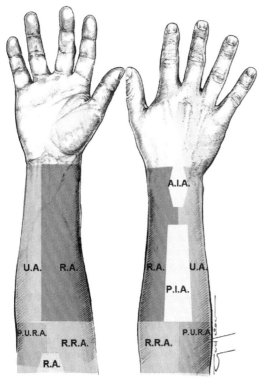

Fig. 1. Vascular territories of the forearm. AIA, anterior interosseous artery; BA, brachial artery; PIA, posterior interosseous artery; PURA, posterior ulnar recurrent artery; RA, radial artery; RRA, radial recurrent artery; UA, ulnar artery.

Although for the pedicled flaps, due to their large rotation axis, the major indication is represented by coverage of defects located on the dorsal aspect of the hand, on the first web space, and on the thumb, the transposition flaps can cover tissue forearm and elbow defects.[8]

- It is easier to detect proximal perforators with Doppler examination because of smaller perforators in the distal area because they are more superficial and can interfere with the Doppler signal.
- Each arterial perforator is accompanied by one or two venae comitantes with communicating branches between them to build a very rich venous plexus that drains into the superficial and the deep systems of veins.

LATERAL ARM PERFORATOR FLAP

The first description of the lateral arm flap was by Song and coworkers[9] 1982 as a free microvascular flap for defect coverage in head and neck.

Vascular Anatomy

The intermuscular septum perforators originate from two main branches in the middle of the upper arm between the acromion and the lateral epicondyle from the profunda brachial artery. These main branches are the anterior and posterior radial collateral arteries. The posterior radial collateral artery is the nourishing artery for the lateral arm flap.[10] The posterior radial collateral artery originates in the radial groove of the humerus and has a diameter of 2 mm at its proximal origin.[11] Along its course within the lateral intermuscular septum, the posterior radial collateral artery gives rise to four to five septocutaneous perforators (1–15 cm proximal to the lateral epicondyle).[11,12] The most constant perforator can be found about 9 cm above the lateral epicondyle.[13] The posterior radial collateral artery communicates with a rich vascular plexus that extends well into the proximal forearm for the extended lateral arm flap.[14]

Flap Harvesting

The longitudinal flap is centered over a line running from the deltoid insertion to the lateral epicondyle of the humerus. This axis runs along the lateral intermuscular septum of the upper arm where the dominant pedicle of the flap—the posterior radial collateral artery with its two venae comitantes—is found. The lower lateral cutaneous or the posterior cutaneous nerve of the forearm can also be harvested with the flap and used as a vascularized nerve graft.

The lateral arm flap can be used as an adipofascial or free fascial flap when very thin and pliable coverage is required. Also, the flap can harvested as an osteocutaneous flap with parts of the lateral humerus. One or two branches of the posterior collateral artery directly and constantly supplying the bone between 2 to 7 cm proximal to the lateral epicondyle can be included in flap harvest.[15] Depending on flap positioning, the overall pedicle length can reach up to 11 cm with the artery having a diameter of 2 to 2.5 mm at its proximal origin from brachial artery.[10]

Inclusion of the distal plexus allows the lateral arm flap to be extended up to 12 cm beyond the lateral epicondyle or the proximal forearm skin.[14] Depending on the patient's body habitus, the donor site can be closed primarily in the majority of cases if flap width is limited to 6 to 7 cm.[16] A case presentation figured out with a perforator flap for covering a forearm tumor defect is demonstrated (**Fig. 3**).

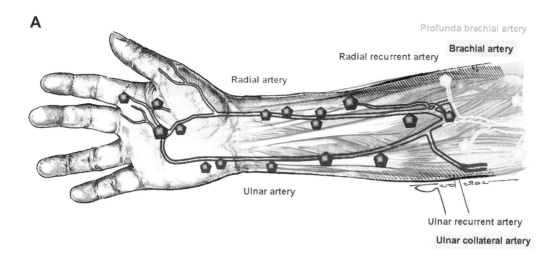

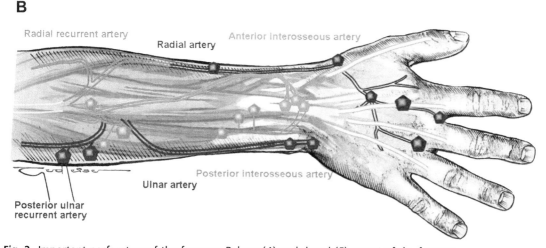

Fig. 2. Important perforators of the forearm. Palmar (*A*) and dorsal (*B*) aspect of the forearm.

POSTERIOR INTEROSSEOUS ARTERY PERFORATOR FLAP

The first description of the posterior interosseous artery flap was by Zancolli and Angrigiani[17] and Penteado and colleagues.[18] Zancolli and Angrigiani[17] used the posterior interosseous artery flap mainly for treating severe adduction contractures of the thumb.

Vascular Anatomy

The posterior interosseous artery originates in most of the cases from the common interosseous artery and infrequently from the ulnar artery.[18] It courses distally on the septum between the muscle (M) extensor digiti minimi and the M extensor carpi ulnaris.[19,20] The posterior interosseous artery comes up through the abductor pollicis longus muscle belly at the junction of the proximal and middle third of the forearm.[21] The perforating arteries run perpendicular to the skin and fan out in all directions.[22] Usually three perforators can be detected on the dorsal ulnar side of the middle third of the forearm [see **Fig. 2**]. The perforators, after piercing the fascia, form a suprafascial vascular network.[21] After its emergence in the back of the forearm, the posterior interosseous artery has an average external caliber of 1.6 mm (range 0.9 to 2.7 mm), whereas the anastomotic branch to the anterior interosseous artery has a caliber of 0.7 mm (range 0.2 to 1.2 mm).[18]

Anastomoses in the distal area of the forearm to the anterior interosseous artery, at the level of the ulnar head, enable the harvest of the posterior

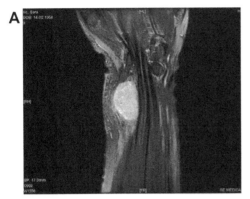

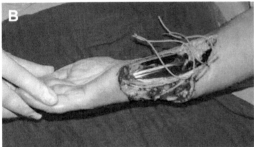

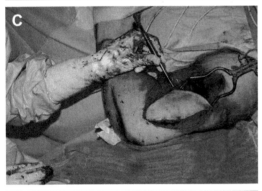

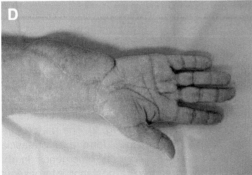

Fig. 3. (*A*) MRI scan of a female patient with a synovial cell sarcoma of the wrist-distal forearm. (*B*) Lateral arm perforator flap for defect coverage of the forearm. Defect at the palmar ulnar aspect of the forearm after resection of the sarcoma. (*C*) Harvesting of the lateral arm flap. (*D*) Postoperative result.

interosseous artery perforator flap as a retrograde-based island flap.[18] This anastomosis is very consistent and lies approximately 5 cm proximal to the ulnar styloid at the proximal edge of the pronator quadratus muscle.[17,20,21] The posterior interosseous artery runs distally to the proximal edge of the extensor retinaculum. This site is the most distal pivot point of the reversed pedicled posterior interosseous perforator flap.

Flap Harvesting

The course of the artery corresponds to a line drawn from the radial epicondyle to the distal radioulnar joint. The flap must be designed to involve the perforators of the skin in the middle third of the posterior forearm on the dorsoulnar side. The skin incision starts at the level of the distal anastomosis between the two interosseous arteries and continues along the radial side of the flap in the distal forearm.[17]

The average length of the pedicle is 7.1 cm.[20] The first medium-sized perforator gives the distal limit of the flap and is an average 7.4 cm above the wrist joint.[20] The posterior interosseous artery may become very small as it travels distally in approximately 6% of the cases.[19] Venous congestion may be possible[19] and, therefore, elevation of the flap with a cutaneous vein is recommended for venous supercharging if this is technically possible.[21]

ULNAR ARTERY PERFORATOR FLAP

The first description of the ulnar forearm flap, mainly for coverage of head and neck defects, was by Lovie and colleagues.[23] Becker and Gilbert[24] described the dorsal ulnar flap, which is based on the dorsal ulnar artery.

Vascular Anatomy

The ulnar artery gives perforators in the proximal and distal area. However, the most important are in the distal area.

Two to four fasciocutaneous perforators originate from the proximal ulnar artery. The first perforator is located approximately 1 cm from the origin of the ulnar artery and the others are located 3 to 5 cm from the origin at 0.6- to 0.9-cm intervals (approximate diameter is 0.3–0.8 mm).[25] They reach the surface by passing along the fascial septum between M flexor carpi ulnaris and M flexor digitorum superficialis.[25]

The dorsal branch of the ulnar artery emerges about 4 cm proximal to the pisiform between the flexor carpi ulnaris muscle and the M flexor digitorum superficialis. The ulnar dorsal artery runs dorsally and distally under the flexor carpi ulnaris muscle.[26] After 3 to 6 cm of a common trunk, the dorsal ulnar artery branches off three ways: proximal, medial, and distal.[24] The proximal branch enters the flexor carpi ulnaris muscle at 4 to 6 cm from its tendinous insertion of the pisiform bone. The medial branch divides into ascending and descending branches. The ascending branch divides into multiple ramifications. It provides the vascularization of a large area of skin on the ulnar side of the forearm.[24]

The descending branch passes in the opposite direction and is accompanied by the dorsal branch of the ulnar nerve. It provides the vascular supply to the skin area over the three ulnar metacarpal bones and the hypothenar eminence.[24] The distal branch nourishes the os pisiforme. The diameter of the dorsal branch is 0.9 to 1.8 mm at its origin from the ulnar artery.[27] They fan out in all directions and anastomose longitudinally.[2,3] Becker and Gilbert[24] reported the absence of the dorsal branch of the ulnar artery in 2% of dissections. In approximately 7%, the dorsal branch arises from the artery interossea anterior.[28]

Flap Harvesting

Proximal ulnar perforator flap

The ulnar fascial-based perforator flap was described by El-Khatib and colleagues[25] based on the proximal perforators of the ulnar artery. The flap should incorporate at least two perforators at its base. An incision is centered along the longitudinal axis of the flap and deepened to the subdermis. It is important to preserve one lobule of fat to keep the subdermal plexus intact. Flap dissection starts at the distal end, goes toward the proximal end, and includes both the deep fascia and the subcutaneous tissue. The pivot point of the flap is usually 4 to 5 cm distal to the elbow joint. The flap is then rotated to cover the defect over the cubital region and immediately skin grafted. The donor site defect can be closed directly under most circumstances.[25]

Distal ulnar perforator flap

The flap is outlined on the dorsoulnar aspect of the distal forearm and located close to the ulnar head. The skin is incised longitudinally on the palmar aspect of the forearm. The incision lies over the flexor carpi ulnaris tendon. On the dorsal aspect it lies between the fourth and fifth extensor digitorum. The cutaneous artery is localized as it emerges under the flexor carpi ulnaris with the dorsal branch of the ulnar nerve. The flap is harvested in a proximal to distal direction. A large superficial vein should be

incorporated into the flap. The flap can also be harvested as a fascial flap. The donor site is closed mainly in most cases. A case presentation figured out with a distal ulnar perforator flap for covering a palmar hand defect is demonstrated in **Fig. 4**.

RADIAL ARTERY PERFORATOR FLAP

The radial forearm flap was originally described as a free flap by Yang and colleagues[29] in 1981.

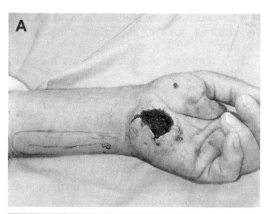

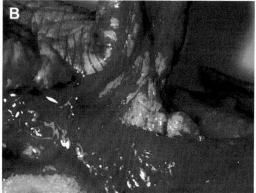

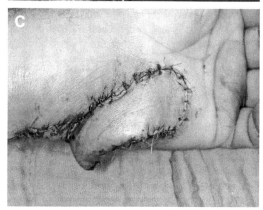

Fig. 4. (A) A distal ulnar perforator flap for covering a palmar ulnar-sided hand defect. (B) Preoperative planning perforator. (C) Postoperative aspect.

Vascular Anatomy

The radial artery courses between the brachioradialis and the flexor carpi radialis muscles to the radial styloid process in the forearm. The radial artery supplies the major part of the forearm (see **Fig. 1**). The mean number of branches of the radial artery that reach the fascial plane is approximately 20 (range 15–25), with a mean diameter of 0.6 mm (range 0.3–0.9 mm). In the proximal forearm, the vessels are less numerous but larger in diameter than in the distal forearm.[4] At least three relatively large perforators existed in all clinical cases, with at least one large perforator located in each of the proximal, middle, and distal thirds of the forearm.[30]

Three territories of perforators are important (see **Fig. 2**):

1. Proximal area. The inferior cubital artery perforator, the largest perforator (0.5 to 1.0 mm diameter), emerges from the fascia between the brachioradialis and pronator teres muscles. The origin of this vessel and its surface-marking varies from 2.0 to 5 cm. (average 4 cm) below the mid point of interepicondylar on the anterior aspect of the forearm.[6]
2. Middle area. Few muscular and septocutaneous perforators emerge in the proximal two thirds of the forearm.
3. Distal area. The distal perforators are smaller (0.3–0.9 mm) than the proximal one. They emerge between 2 and 7 cm above the radial styloid between the brachioradialis muscle and the flexor carpi radialis muscle area.[2]

Flap Harvesting

Proximal radial artery perforator flap
The proximal radial artery perforator flap is raised from the antebrachial surface. Ligature of distal perforators is required to enhance the arc of rotation of the flap. The skin island of the flap is located at the middle third of the forearm palmar surface. The pivot point of the flap is located 5 cm from the interepicondylar line.[4]

Reversed forearm radial artery perforator flap
Flap elevation is initiated from the lateral margin to identify the septocutaneous perforators. The medial border of the flap is incised and the flap is islanded completely. The superficial radial nerve and deep fascia should be preserved. The perforator vessels should be dissected along their course to the radial artery in the lateral intermuscular septum. After that, the proximal portions of the radial vessel can be ligated and cut for distally based pedicled flap transfer.[30,31]

Free radial artery perforator flap
The flap is elevated as a distal row perforator-based fasciocutaneous flap with a very short segment of the radial artery. The venous outflow is provided by the cephalic vein.[32]

INTRINSIC HAND FLAPS
Dorsal Ulnar Thumb Flap

Vascular anatomy
The princeps pollicis artery arises from the radial artery in the first web space, travels on the palmar surface of the thumb at the level of the metacarpophalangeal joint flexion crease, and divides into the ulnar and radial digital arteries. The dorsal of the thumb skin has an independent blood supply. It originates from the princeps pollicis artery and travels longitudinally along the dorsal ulnar surface of the thumb. The artery is very constant.[33] The dorsal collateral ulnar artery can be found an average distance of 1.4 cm ulnar to the median axis of the thumb at the head of the first metacarpal bone, and 1 cm ulnar to the median axis of the thumb at the head of the proximal phalanx.[33] Two communications are important: the proximal one communicates with the ulnar palmar digital at the neck of the proximal phalanx and the second one communicates with the proximal nail fold arcade.

Flap harvesting
The flap is harvested over the dorsal aspect of the metacarpophalangeal joint, centered over the dorsal ulnar collateral artery. A Doppler examination is mandatory. The flap is raised in a proximal to distal direction. The pedicle is not skeletonized and should be harvested with a 1 cm cuff of surrounding soft tissue. The donor site can be closed mainly or with a full-thickness skin graft.[33] Similar to the dorsal ulnar thumb flap, a dorsal radial thumb flap can be used for defect coverage at the thumb.[34] A case presentation figured out with a reversed dorsal radial thumb flap for covering a thumb defect is shown in **Fig. 5**.

First Dorsal Metacarpal Artery Flap (Kite Flap Proximally Pedicled)

A flap from the dorsum of the index finger was already used for thumb reconstruction by Hilgenfeldt[35] and a similar island flap with a cutaneous pedicle was reported by Holevich.[36] Later, Foucher and Braun's[37] modification of the Holevich flap ("kite flap") was introduced as a routine procedure.

Vascular anatomy
The dorsal metacarpal arteries supply the dorsal proximal portion of the hand while the dorsal

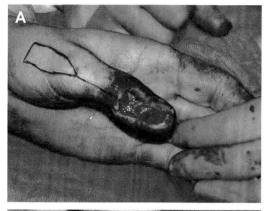

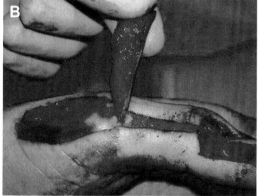

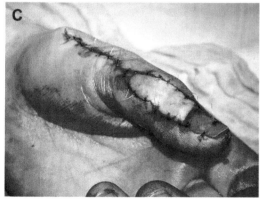

Fig. 5. A reverse dorsal radial thumb flap is used for coverage of a dorsal defect at the thumb. (*A*) Preoperative planning. (*B*) Flap harvesting. (*C*) Postoperative aspect.

perforating metacarpal arterial branches of the deep palmar arch supply the dorsal distal hand and proximal dorsal fingers.[38]

The first dorsal metacarpal artery (FDMA) originates from the radial artery or, less frequently, from the dorsal superficial antebrachial artery.[37] The FDMA travels parallel to the dorsal surface of the second metacarpal and superficial to the first dorsal interosseus muscle. The FDMA anastomoses at the level of the metacarpal neck with

dorsal perforating branches from the palmar metacarpal arteries.[39] This anastomosis is important for the reversed island flap.

The FDMA constantly gives three fascial branches: a radial branch, an ulnar branch, and an intermediate branch. The radial branch of the FDMA runs along the dorsum of the first metacarpal bone. The ulnar branch of the FDMA courses over the second metacarpal up to the index metacarpophalangeal joint. The Intermediate branch of the FDMA runs toward the first web space.[40]

Flap harvesting

The FDMA flap is elevated from distal to proximal and begins by incising the flap over the dorsal proximal phalanx just above the paratenon layer. One or more subcutaneous veins and a small branch of the superficial radial nerve[41] should be incorporated into the flap. The dissection of the flap includes the first dorsal interosseous muscle fascia, because the nourishing vessel lies just beneath the fascia.[42] The pedicle should not be skeletonized and can be raised with a cuff of fibrofatty tissue. The flap can be extended by including nearly the entire dorsum of the index finger including the distal interphalangeal joint and the skin covering the metacarpophalangeal joint.[43] The FDMA supplies the dorsal skin of the proximal phalanx. Inclusion of the skin of the middle phalanx is randomly patterned. Vascularized periosteum or tendon can also be raised with the flap.[42] The donor site at the index finger is covered with a full-thickness skin graft.

Second Dorsal Metacarpal Artery Flap

Vascular anatomy

The second dorsal metacarpal artery (SDMA) originates from the dorsal carpal arch or, less frequently, from the deep palmar arch, the FDMA, anterior interosseous artery, or the radial artery.[44] The SDMA courses beneath the extensor tendons and then superficial to the second dorsal interosseous muscle. The SDMA ramified at the level of the metacarpal heads and the branches travels to the proximal dorsal phalanx of the index and the middle finger where they anastomized with the dorsal branches of the palmar digital arteries.[44] One or more larger perforators can be found between the second and third metacarpal heads in the second intermetacarpal space.

Flap harvesting

The flap is incised circumferentially and dissected off the extensor tendon paratenon from the proximal phalanx in a distal to proximal fashion. To safeguard the artery, the dorsal interosseous fascia must be included with the pedicle over the full width of the muscle. It is not necessary to identify the artery itself.[45]

An extended version of the SDMA flap is possible but if the flap is extended beyond the proximal interphalangeal joint, distal flap necrosis or donor site difficulties may occur.[45]

Reverse Dorsal Metacarpal Artery Flap

Vascular anatomy
The presence of distal intermetacarpal anastomoses between dorsal and palmar vascular networks makes it possible to raise distally based cutaneous island flaps oriented along the axis of the dorsal metacarpal arteries.[46,47] The dorsal carpal arch is formed by the carpal branches of

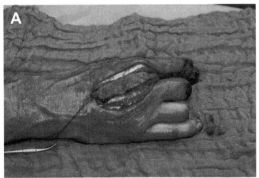

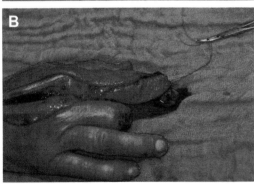

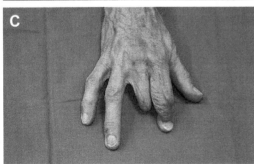

Fig. 6. An extended reverse SDMA flap for coverage of a distal dorsal index finger defect is demonstrated. (*A, B*) Flap harvesting. (*C*) Postoperative aspect.

the radial and ulnar arteries with contributions from both the anterior and posterior interosseous arteries.[48]

The first dorsal metacarpal artery comes with a direct branch from the radial artery. The second, third, and fourth dorsal metacarpal arteries arise from the dorsal carpal arch.[49] The tendons of the extensor digitorum communis cover the proximal two thirds of the second to the fourth dorsal metacarpal arteries.

Flap harvesting
The flap can be raised on the second, third, or fourth intermetacarpal spaces (fashioned as an ellipse).The axis of rotation of the flap corresponds to the site where the recurrent cutaneous branch of the dorsal metacarpal vessel enters the skin. This is usually 0.5 to 1 cm proximal to the adjacent metacarpophalangeal joint.[49]

The skin is incised on one side of the ellipse down to the paratenon of the extensor tendon. It is then undermined from the proximal area with care. The pedicle is identified distally to the intertendinous connection of the corresponding intermetacarpal space.[49,50] A case presentation figured out with an extended reverse dorsal metacarpal artery flap, described by Pelissier and colleagues,[51] for covering a thumb defect is shown in **Fig. 6**.

REFERENCES

1. Blondeel PN, Van Landuyt KH, Monstrey SJ, et al. The "Gent" consensus on perforator flap terminology: preliminary definitions. Plast Reconstr Surg 2003;112(5):1378–83.
2. Georgescu AV, Matei I, Ardelean F, et al. Microsurgical nonmicrovascular flaps in forearm and hand reconstruction. Microsurgery 2007;27(5):384–94.
3. Kanellakos GW, Yang D, Morris SF. Cutaneous vasculature of the forearm. Ann Plast Surg 2003; 50:387.
4. Tiengo C, Macchi V, Porzionato A, et al. Anatomical study of perforator arteries in the distally based radial forearm fasciosubcutaneous flap. Clin Anat 2004;17:636–42.
5. Morris SF, Taylor GI. Predicting the survival of experimental skin flaps with the knowledge of the vascular architecture. Plast Reconstr Surg 1993;92:1352–61.
6. Lamberty BGH, Cormack GC. The forearm angiotomes. Br J Plast Surg 1982;35:420.
7. Inoue Y, Taylor GI. The angiosomes of the forearm: anatomic study and clinical implications. Plast Reconstr Surg 1996;98:195–210.
8. Matei I, Georgescu A, Chiroiu B, et al. Harvesting of forearm perforator flaps based on intraoperative

vascular exploration: clinical experiences and litera-ture review. Microsurgery 2008;28(5):321–30.

9. Song R, Song Y, Yu Y, et al. The upper arm free flap. Clin Plast Surg 1982;9:27–35.

10. Sauerbier M, Giessler GA. The free lateral arm flap for hand and wrist coverage. In: Cooney WP, Moran SL, editors. Master techniques in orthopedic surgery: soft tissue. Philadelphia: Lippincott Wil-liams & Wilkins; 2008. p. 179–89.

11. Yousif NJ, Warren R, Matloub HS, et al. The lateral arm fascial free flap: its anatomy and use in reconstruction. Plast Reconstr Surg 1990;86(6): 1138–45.

12. Chen HC, el-Gammal TA. The lateral arm fascial free flap for resurfacing of the hand and fingers. Plast Reconstr Surg 1997;99(2):454–9.

13. Hwang K, Lee WJ, Jung CY, et al. Cutaneous perfo-rators of the upper arm and clinical applications. J Reconstr Microsurg 2005;21(7):463–9.

14. Brandt KE, Khouri RK. The lateral arm/proximal fore-arm flap. Plast Reconstr Surg 1993;92(6):1137–43.

15. Haas F, Rappl T, Koch H, et al. Free osteocutaneous lateral arm flap: anatomy and clinical applications. Microsurgery 2003;23(2):87–95.

16. Scheker LR, Lister GD, Wolff TW. The lateral arm free flap in releasing severe contracture of the first web space. J Hand Surg 1988;1:146–50.

17. Zancolli EA, Angrigiani C. Posterior interosseous island forearm flap. J Hand Surg Br 1988;13(2):130–5.

18. Penteado CV, Masquelet AC, Chevrel JP. The anatomic basis of the fascio-cutaneous flap of the posterior interosseous artery. Surg Radiol Anat 1986;8(4):209–15.

19. Büchler U, Frey HP. Retrograde posterior inteross-eous flap. J Hand Surg Am 1991;16(2):283–92.

20. Bayon P, Pho RW. Anatomical basis of dorsal fore-arm flap. Based on posterior interosseous vessels. J Hand Surg Br 1988;13(4):435–9.

21. Shibata M. Posterior interosseous artery perforator flap. In: Blondeel PM, Hallock GG, Morris SF, et al, editors. Perforator flaps. St Louis: Quality Medical Publishing; 2006. p. 270–82.

22. Manchot C. The cutaneous arteries of the human body. New York: Springer-Verlag; 1983.

23. Lovie MJ, Duncan GM, Glasson DW. The ulnar artery forearm free flap. Br J Plast Surg 1984;37(4): 486–92.

24. Becker C, Gilbert A. The ulnar flap-description and application. Eur J Plast Surg 1988;11:79–82.

25. El-Khatib HA, Mahboub TA, Ali TA. Use of an adipo-fascial flap based on the proximal perforators of the ulnar artery to correct contracture of elbow burn scars: an anatomic and clinical approach. Plast Re-constr Surg 2002;109(1):130–6.

26. Vergara-Amador E. Anatomical study of the ulnar dorsal artery and design of a new retrograde ulnar dorsal flap. Plast Reconstr Surg 2008;121:1716–23.

27. Yang D, Morris SF. Ulnar artery perforator flap. In: Blondeel PM, Hallock GG, Morris SF, et al, editors. Perforator flaps. St Louis: Quality Medical Publishing; 2006. p. 284–99.

28. Bertelli JA, Pagliei A. The neurocutaneous flap based on the dorsal branches of the ulnar artery and nerve: a new flap for extensive reconstruction of the hand. Plast Reconstr Surg 1998;101:1537–43.

29. Yang G, Chen B, Gao Y. The forearm free skin flap transplantation. Natl Med J China 1981;61:139–41.

30. Mateev MA, Ogawa R, Trunov L, et al. Shape-modified radial artery perforator flap method: analysis of 112 cases. Plast Reconstr Surg 2009;123(5):1533–43.

31. Yang D, Morris SF. Radial artery perforator flap. In: Blondeel PM, Hallock GG, Morris SF, et al, editors. Perforator flaps. St Louis: Quality Medical Publishing; 2006. p. 301–17.

32. Safak T, Akyürek M. Free transfer of the radial fore-arm flap with preservation of the radial artery. Ann Plast Surg 2000;45:97–9.

33. Brunelli F, Vigasio A, Valenti P, et al. Arterial anatomy and clinical application of the dorsoulnar flap of the thumb. J Hand Surg Am 1999;24(4):803–11.

34. Moschella F, Cordova A. Reverse homodigital dorsal radial flap of the thumb. Plast Reconstr Surg 2006; 117(3):920–6.

35. Hilgenfeldt O. Operativer Daumenersatz. Stuttgart: Enke Verlag; 1950.

36. Holevich J. A new method of restoring sensibility to the thumb. J Bone Joint Surg Br 1963;45:496–502.

37. Foucher G, Braun JB. A new island flap transfer from the dorsum of the index to the thumb. Plast Reconstr Surg 1979;63(3):344–9.

38. Yang D, Morris SF. Vascular basis of dorsal digital and metacarpal skin flaps. J Hand Surg Am 2001; 26(1):142–6.

39. Germann G, Hornung R, Raff T. Two new applica-tions for the first dorsal metacarpal artery pedicle in the treatment of severe hand injuries. J Hand Surg Br 1995;20(4):525–8.

40. Sherif MM. First dorsal metacarpal artery flap in hand reconstruction. I. Anatomical study. J Hand Surg Am 1994;19(1):26–31.

41. Small JO, Brennen MD. The first dorsal metacarpal artery neurovascular island flap. J Hand Surg Br 1988;13(2):136–45.

42. Sherif MM. First dorsal metacarpal artery flap in hand reconstruction. II. Clinical application. J Hand Surg Am 1994;19(1):32–8.

43. Gebhard B, Meissl G. An extended first dorsal meta-carpal artery neurovascular island flap. J Hand Surg Br 1995;20(4):529–31.

44. Earley MJ, Milner RH. Dorsal metacarpal flaps. Br J Plast Surg 1987;40(4):333–41.

45. Earley MJ. The second dorsal metacarpal artery neurovascular island flap. J Hand Surg Br 1989; 14(4):434–40.

46. Dautel G, Merle M. Dorsal metacarpal reverse flaps. Anatomical basis and clinical application. J Hand Surg Br 1991;16(4):400–5.

47. Levame JH, Otero C, Berdugo G. Arterial vascularization of teguments of the dorsal surface of the hand and fingers. Ann Chir Plast 1967;12(4):316–24.

48. Coleman SS, Anson BJ. Arterial patterns in the hand based upon a study of 650 specimens. Surg Gynecol Obstet 1961;113:409–24.

49. Quaba AA, Davison PM. The distally-based dorsal hand flap. Br J Plast Surg 1990;43(1):28–39.

50. Dautel G, Merle M. Direct and reverse dorsal metacarpal flaps. Br J Plast Surg 1992;45(2): 123–30.

51. Pelissier P, Casoli V, Bakhach J, et al. Reverse dorsal digital and metacarpal flaps: a review of 27 cases. Plast Reconstr Surg 1999;103(1): 159–65.

Versatility of the Pedicled Anterolateral Thigh Flap

Peter C. Neligan, MB, BCh, FRCS(I), FRCS(C), FACS[a],*,
Declan A. Lannon, MB, MSc, FRCS(Plast)[b]

KEYWORDS

- Pedicled flap • Anterolateral thigh flap • Flap harvest
- Flap transposition

Since it was first described by Song and colleagues[1] in 1984, the anterolateral thigh flap has been more commonly used as a free flap than as a pedicled flap. However, it is extremely useful as a pedicled flap and can be used to reconstruct a wide variety of defects in the pelvis, the perineum, and the lower abdomen.[2–4] For these purposes, the flap is pedicled on proximal flow from the descending branch of the lateral circumflex femoral artery. Distally based pedicled anterolateral thigh flaps are described[5–7] but are not discussed other than to caution that venous outflow can sometimes be a problem with this particular configuration. However, they have been used successfully in the coverage of defects around the knee and the lower leg.[8,9] Here the authors describe the use of the proximally based anterolateral thigh flap for reconstruction of perineal, pelvic, and lower abdominal defects. This article reviews the major applications of the proximally pedicled anterolateral thigh flap, describes the technique of flap harvest, and discusses techniques for flap transposition as well as pointing out some potential hazards.

VASCULAR ANATOMY

The vascular anatomy of the anterolateral thigh flap has been well described.[10,11] It is important to note, however, that one side of the body is not a mirror image of the other and, as with other perforator flaps, a case can be made for preoperative

imaging.[12,13] The blood supply comes from the descending branch of the lateral circumflex femoral artery. An ascending or transverse branch supplies the tensor fascia lata muscle and the skin overlying that muscle. The descending branch runs between vastus lateralis laterally and rectus femoris medially. The overlying skin is supplied, for the most part, by intramuscular perforators that usually run through vastus lateralis and less frequently through rectus femoris. Perforators supplying the flap usually penetrate the anterior aspect of the vastus lateralis (**Fig. 1**). In less than 15% of cases, the perforators run in the septum between the 2 muscles.[14] In this situation no intramuscular dissection is required. The configuration of the perforators has been described by Yu and Youssef.[11] They describe A, B, and C perforators, with A being proximal and C distal to perforator B. The nerve to vastus lateralis runs alongside the main pedicle. Care must be taken during dissection to ensure that the nerve is not injured.

FLAP DESIGN

A line is drawn from the anterior superior iliac spine to the lateral border of the patella (**Fig. 2**). This line represents the surface marking of the septum between vastus lateralis and rectus femoris. The midportion of this line marks the site at which the perforators are most likely to be encountered and detected. The authors' preference is to use a hand-held Doppler to locate the perforators,

[a] Center for Reconstructive Surgery, University of Washington Medical Center, 1959 NE Pacific Street, Box 356410, Seattle, WA 98195-6410, USA
[b] The Ulster Hospital, Dundonald, Belfast, Northern Ireland, United Kingdom
* Corresponding author. Center for Reconstructive Surgery, University of Washington Medical Center, 1959 NE Pacific Street, Box 356410, Seattle, WA 98195-6410.
E-mail address: pneligan@u.washington.edu

Clin Plastic Surg 37 (2010) 677–681
doi:10.1016/j.cps.2010.07.001
0094-1298/10/$ — see front matter © 2010 Elsevier Inc. All rights reserved.

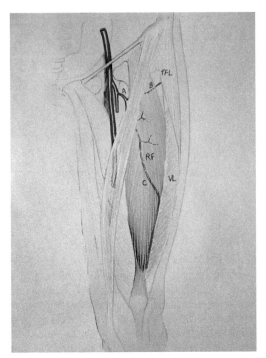

Fig. 1. The lateral circumflex artery (A), a branch of the profunda femoris, has a lateral (ascending) branch (B) that supplies the tensor fasciae lata muscle (TFL) and a descending branch (C) that supplies the anterolateral thigh flap. This vessels runs under rectus femoris (RF) and then in the septum, between rectus femoris and vastus lateralis (VL).

recognizing that this method may not always be accurate.[15] The flap can be raised to include any of the elements supplied by the vasculature. It can incorporate muscle (vastus lateralis), fascia, and skin. The choice of which tissues to include will be dictated by the reconstructive requirements. The technique may be modified accordingly. For many of the reconstructive applications that a pedicled anterolateral thigh flap can address in the lower abdomen, the fascial element of the

flap can be important, which is particularly the case when reconstructing through abdominal wall defects. Often, the amount of fascia required is larger than the amount of skin required. If this is the case, an excess of fascia over skin can easily be harvested (**Fig. 3**). Vascularized fascia lata in abdominal wall reconstruction is said to have the advantage of preventing adhes between the fascia and the abdominal viscera.[16] If no fascia is required for the reconstruction, then a skin-only flap can be designed and the fascia simply incised around the perforators (**Fig. 4**). Furthermore, if muscle is a required element of the reconstruction, the flap can be raised as a myocutaneous flap incorporating the vastus lateralis muscle. The technique of dissection will depend on what elements are being included with the flap. The dimensions of the flap will obviously be dictated by the size of the defect to be reconstructed. However, the vascular pedicle of the anterolateral thigh can carry a large flap (up to 30 cm). To perfuse such a large skin paddle, however, more than 1 perforator may need to be harvested with the flap. If multiple perforators are available, it is judicious to sequentially clamp them so as to ensure that the selected perforators will perfuse the flap (see **Fig. 4**). Pedicle length can also be particularly important when the flap is being designed as a pedicled flap; the longer the pedicle, the greater the arc of rotation. Preoperative imaging may be particularly helpful when planning a pedicled anterolateral thigh flap because the location of the perforator has a bearing on pedicle length and, therefore, on the arc of rotation of the flap. A distally placed perforator, the C perforator according to Yu's classification, can add considerable length and can be chosen if it is of appropriate size. The more distal perforators, however, tend to

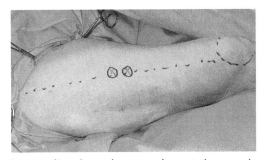

Fig. 2. A line drawn between the anterior superior iliac spine and the lateral border of the patella is the surface marking of the septum between rectus femoris and vastus lateralis. The midportion of this line is where perforators will be found.

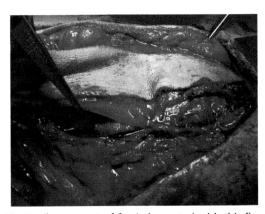

Fig. 3. The amount of fascia harvested with this flap exceeds the amount of skin. This picture shows the excess thigh fascia being sutured to the abdominal wall fascia.

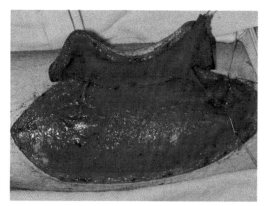

Fig. 4. In this suprafascial flap dissection, 2 perforators have been isolated. A microvascular clamp has been placed on the proximal perforator to ensure that the distal perforator can perfuse the whole flap.

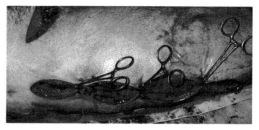

Fig. 5. Penetrating towel clamps are used to temporarily approximate the wound edges to facilitate closure. If closure is this tight, it is important to ensure that patients are in a fit condition to report symptoms of compartment syndrome.

have a longer intramuscular course. Although the extra pedicle length gained from dissecting these perforators may be desirable, the amount of intramuscular dissection can be an important issue. Regardless of the position of the perforator, size is important and the perforator needs clinical evaluation to ensure that it can adequately perfuse the flap. As already mentioned, if ever there is any doubt, sequentially clamping the perforators (see **Fig. 4**) can be a good way to determine which perforator offers the best perfusion.

The width of the flap is also important because it will determine whether or not the donor site will need a skin graft or whether it can be closed by direct approximation. Direct closure is desirable because a skin graft in this area is unsightly and not always well tolerated by patients. Although it is generally accepted that a width of 8 cm can usually be closed directly, it has been the authors' experience that much wider defects can be closed directly. If the flap does not contain fascia, it is generally much easier to close the donor defect than when the fascia has been harvested with the flap because the fascia contains and constrains the thigh musculature, which, when fascia has been harvested with the flap, tends to bulge and make closure more difficult. Regardless of whether or not fascia has been harvested with the flap, penetrating towel clamps can be used to temporarily approximate the wound edges (**Fig. 5**) allowing sufficient tissue creep to facilitate closure. Care must be exercised, however, in situations where patients are unable to report symptoms that might indicate too tight a closure. The authors have encountered 2 cases of compartment syndrome, in the presence of epidural anesthesia, that was caused by a closure that was too tight.[17]

ARC OF ROTATION

The proximally pedicled anterolateral thigh flap will easily reach the lower abdomen and perineum.[2,18–20] As already mentioned, choosing a more distal perforator increases the length of the pedicle and, therefore, the arc of rotation. However, size is important when choosing an appropriate perforator. Choosing a distal perforator simply because of position and not because of size is not advised. The arc of rotation is also determined by the method by which the flap is transferred. The lateral circumflex femoral artery is a branch of the profunda femoris. The artery comes off the lateral aspect of the profunda at a point that is medial to the proximal segment of the rectus femoris muscle. It runs under that muscle and eventually runs between the rectus femoris and vastus lateralis muscles. To dissect the pedicle to its origin, the rectus femoris must be retracted. Tunneling the flap under the rectus femoris (**Fig. 6**) increases its arc of rotation and allows the flap to reach the perineum and lower abdomen. For more lateral defects of the lower abdomen or thigh, tunneling under rectus femoris offers no advantage. In fact it may shorten the arc of rotation in that direction. Sometimes dividing the main pedicle to rectus femoris, as the flap is tunneled under this muscle, will significantly increase the arc of rotation. However, caution is required in relation to these maneuvers because ischemic damage to the rectus femoris muscle may result from division of its main pedicle,[21] and denervation may result from tunneling under its proximal third because it is innervated by 2 to 4 nerve branches entering posteromedially in this region.[22]

In addition, the saphenous vein is at risk during medial subcutaneous tunnelling.[23] If rectus femoris pedicle ligation is being considered intraoperatively, it is prudent to clamp the pedicle and observe for muscle vascularity before pedicle division. The donor site is closed primarily in layers or

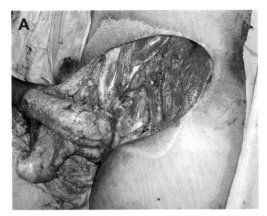

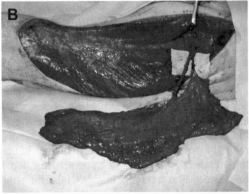

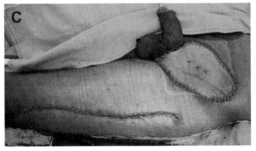

Fig. 6. (*A*) Defect following radical excision of metastatic carcinoma to the groin. (*B*) A tunnel is created under rectus femoris through which the flap can be passed. (*C*) Flap inset into lower abdominal defect.

by using a split-thickness skin graft depending on the width of the flap harvested and patient characteristics. Primary closure of the fascia is required if suprafascial flap harvesting has been performed to prevent muscle hernia, which can be painful. In the authors' experience, the arc of rotation extends to the lower costal margin, the posterior superior iliac spine, the trochanteric area, the anterior margin of anus, and the contralateral iliac fossa. Previous reports have indicated that the flap will reach to 8 cm above the umbilicus, the contralateral lower abdomen and inguinal area, the entire groin, and perineum to anus.[24] Gravvanis and colleagues[2]

have also described its use in coverage of a variety of defects.

AVOIDING COMPLICATIONS

Attention to detail can help avoid complications in using this flap. Careful selection of the appropriate perforators is the first step. Care must also be taken to avoid any injury to the pedicle during dissection. As already mentioned, it is important to try to preserve the nerve to vastus lateralis. Judicious division of the pedicle to rectus femoris is important. It is important to avoid tension in the pedicle and not to ask the flap to do too much. If in any doubt, it is easy to convert to a free anterolateral thigh flap. If the flap is being tunneled from the thigh to the area to be reconstructed, it is of prime importance to ensure that the tunnel is wide enough not only to accommodate the flap but also to ensure that the pedicle will not be under any pressure in the immediate postoperative period. This point is particularly important in patients who are obese. The authors' lost 1 flap in an obese patient as the pedicle was avulsed from the flap during passage through a tight tunnel. It is possible to thin the flap,[25] and this may be considered in patients who are obese. However, in the authors' practice, morbid obesity is a relative contraindication for a pedicled anterolateral thigh flap.

SUMMARY

The pedicled anterolateral thigh flap is a useful addition to our armamentarium. It provides excellent cover for defects in the lower abdomen, pelvis, and perineum. It also has the added advantage of not sacrificing any muscle, thereby minimizing the risk for donor morbidity.

REFERENCES

1. Song YG, Chen GZ, Song YL. The free thigh flap: a new free flap concept based on the septocutaneous artery. Br J Plast Surg 1984;37(2):149–59.
2. Gravvanis AI, Tsoutsos DA, Karakitsos D, et al. Application of the pedicled anterolateral thigh flap to defects from the pelvis to the knee. Microsurgery 2006;26(6):432–8.
3. Hallock GG. The proximal pedicled anterolateral thigh flap for lower limb coverage. Ann Plast Surg 2005;55(5):466–9.
4. Wang X, Qiao Q, Burd A, et al. Perineum reconstruction with pedicled anterolateral thigh fasciocutaneous flap. Ann Plast Surg 2006;56(2):151–5.
5. Pan SC, Yu JC, Shieh SJ, et al. Distally based anterolateral thigh flap: an anatomic and clinical study. Plast Reconstr Surg 2004;114(7):1768–75.

6. Heo C, Eun S, Bae R, et al. Distally based anterolateral-thigh (ALT) flap with the aid of multidetector computed tomography. J Plast Reconstr Aesthet Surg 2010;63(5):e465–8.

7. Uygur F, Duman H, Ulkür E, et al. Are reverse flow fasciocutaneous flaps an appropriate option for the reconstruction of severe postburn lower extremity contractures? Ann Plast Surg 2008;61(3):319–24.

8. Lin CH, Hsu CC, Lin CH, et al. Antegrade venous drainage in a reverse-flow anterolateral thigh flap. Plast Reconstr Surg 2009;124(5):273e–4e.

9. Cotrufo S, Hart A. A note of caution on the use of the distally based anterolateral thigh flap: anatomical evidence. Plast Reconstr Surg 2010;125(1):30e–1e.

10. Kawai K, Imanishi N, Nakajima H, et al. Vascular anatomy of the anterolateral thigh flap. Plast Reconstr Surg 2004;114(5):1108–17.

11. Yu P, Youssef A. Efficacy of the handheld Doppler in preoperative identification of the cutaneous perforators in the anterolateral thigh flap. Plast Reconstr Surg 2006;118(4):928–33 [discussion: 934–5].

12. Rozen WM, Ashton MW, Pan WR, et al. Anatomical variations in the harvest of anterolateral thigh flap perforators: a cadaveric and clinical study. Microsurgery 2009;29(1):16–23.

13. Rozen WM, Wagstaff MJ, Grinsell D, et al. The course of anterolateral thigh perforators does not correlate between sides of the body: the role for preoperative imaging. Plast Reconstr Surg 2010; 125(3):132e–4e.

14. Wei FC, Jain V, Celik N, et al. Have we found an ideal soft-tissue flap? An experience with 672 anterolateral thigh flaps. Plast Reconstr Surg 2002;109(7): 2219–26 [discussion: 2227–30].

15. Lin SJ, Rabie A, Yu P. Designing the anterolateral thigh flap without preoperative Doppler or imaging. J Reconstr Microsurg 2009;26(1):67–72.

16. Yildirim S, Taylan G, Akoz T. Use of fascia component of the anterolateral thigh flap for different reconstructive purposes. Ann Plast Surg 2005; 55(5):479–84.

17. Addison PD, Lannon D, Neligan PC. Compartment syndrome after closure of the anterolateral thigh flap donor site: a report of two cases. Ann Plast Surg 2008;60(6):635–8.

18. Descamps MJ, Hayes PM, Hudson DA. Phalloplasty in complete aphallia: pedicled anterolateral thigh flap. J Plast Reconstr Aesthet Surg 2009;62(3): c51 4.

19. Hofer SO. A pedicled anterolateral thigh flap for abdominal reconstruction after previous degloving injury of the donor site: revascularisation of the donor site. Scand J Plast Reconstr Surg Hand Surg 2007;41(4):203–6.

20. Huang LY, Lin H, Liu YT, et al. Anterolateral thigh vastus lateralis myocutaneous flap for vulvar reconstruction after radical vulvectomy: a preliminary experience. Gynecol Oncol 2000;78(3 Pt 1): 391–3.

21. Kimata Y, Uchiyama K, Ebihara S, et al. Anatomic variations and technical problems of the anterolateral thigh flap: a report of 74 cases. Plast Reconstr Surg 1998;102(5):1517–23.

22. Spyriounis PK. The extended approach to the vascular pedicle of the anterolateral thigh perforator flap: anatomical and clinical study. Plast Reconstr Surg 2006;117(3):997–1001 [discussion: 1002–3].

23. Yu P, Sanger JR, Matloub HS, et al. Anterolateral thigh fasciocutaneous island flaps in perineoscrotal reconstruction. Plast Reconstr Surg 2002;109(2): 610–6 [discussion: 617–8].

24. Kimata Y, Uchiyama K, Ebihara S, et al. Anterolateral thigh flap donor-site complications and morbidity. Plast Reconstr Surg 2000;106(3):584–9.

25. Kimura N, Satoh K. Consideration of a thin flap as an entity and clinical applications of the thin anterolateral thigh flap. Plast Reconstr Surg 1996;97(5):985–92.

Perforator Flaps and Supermicrosurgery

Isao Koshima, MD*, Takumi Yamamoto, MD,
Mitsunaga Narushima, MD, Makoto Mihara, MD,
Takuya Iida, MD

KEYWORDS

- Supermicrosurgery • Perforator flaps
- Reconstructive surgery • Supramicrosurgery

WHAT IS SUPERMICROSURGERY OR SUPRAMICROSURGERY?

Supermicrosurgery, or *supramicrosurgery*, is a technique of microneurovascular anastomosis for smaller vessels and single nerve fascicle, and also microneurovascular dissection for these small vessels less than 0.3 to 0.8 mm. This technique needs ultradelicate microsurgical instruments (Emi Company, Swa City, Nagano, Japan) and fain suture materials (Crown Jun Company, Tokyo, Japan) with a needle less than 30 to 80 μm. With this technique, new reconstructive microsurgery using true perforator flaps and nerve flaps has been recently developed.

HISTORY OF SUPERMICROSURGERY

The concept and naming of supermicrosurgery was established in Japan in the 1980s and introduced internationally in 1997.[1] This technique developed a high success rate after replantations above the distal phalanx of the fingers,[2,3] vascularized toenail for finger nail losses,[4] vascularized distal interphalangeal joints, and toe-tip transfers for fingertip reconstructions.[5] In addition, many new free tissue transfers have been developed, including appendix transfer for urethral reconstruction,[6] partial auricular transfer for upper eyelid[7–12] and tracheal loss,[13] toe-web transfers for oral commissure loss,[14] vascularized nerve flaps with perforator vessel,[15] fascicular turnover flaps for nerve gaps,[16] supermicrosurgical

lymphaticovenular anastomosis for obstructive lymphedema in the extremities,[17–19] mini-bone flap, and periosteal flaps.

With this technique, new short T pedicle or true perforator flaps have been developed.[20] These flaps have advantages of short time elevation anywhere in the body. Free perforator-to-perforator flaps are now topic (ie, true perforator flaps with anastomosing small perforators of flap and recipient site <0.8 mm of diameter). Such flaps have been reported as paraumbilical perforator (PUP) adiposal flap or deep inferior epigastric perforator (DIEP) flap for breast reconstruction and facial augmentation,[21–24] thoracodorsal artery perforator (TAP) flap for extremities, anterolateral thigh perforator (ALT) flap for extremities,[20] tensor fasciae lata (TFL) perforator flap for hand, medial thigh perforator flap for foot, gluteal artery perforator flap for facial augmentation,[25] posterior tibial flap for hand coverage, and medial plantar perforator flap for finger pulp coverage.[26–29] Also, vascularized adiposal flaps with these perforators are now useful for facial and breast augmentation.[30]

NEW CLASSIFICATION OF PERFORATOR FLAPS

Based on the authors' previous reports, perforator flaps can be classified as long vascular pedicle perforator flaps (DIEP flaps, ALT and anteromedial thigh [AMT] flaps, TAP flaps); short T pedicle perforator flaps, including a short T-shape segment of large vessels (DIEP or PUP flaps, ALT and AMT

The following are Lecturers in Plastic and Reconstructive Surgery, University of Tokyo: Takumi Yamamoto, Mitsunaga Narushima, Makoto Mihara, Takuya Iida.

Plastic and Reconstructive Surgery, Graduate School of Medicine, University of Tokyo, 7-3-1, Hongo, Bunkyo-ku, Tokyo 113-8655, Japan

* Corresponding author.

E-mail address: koushimai-pla@h.u-tokyo.ac.jp

Clin Plastic Surg 37 (2010) 683–689
doi:10.1016/j.cps.2010.06.009

flaps, TFL flaps, TAP flaps, superficial circumflex iliac artery perforator flaps [SCIP], radial artery perforator flaps, snuff box flaps, medial plantar flaps); and true perforator flaps (**Fig. 1**). The T perforator flaps are usually used as a flow-through perforator flap. The true perforator flap has only perforators and no main trunk vessels.

CASE REPORTS

Representative cases with supermicrosurgical technique are as follows:

Case 1: Distal Phalangeal Replantation

A 47-year-old man amputated the distal phalanx of the left middle finger. Under digital block, the proximal arteriole of digital artery was anastomosed to the distal volar cutaneous venule, and the distal ulnar venule was anastomosed to the proximal cutaneous vein with arteriolar graft as the drainage system. The distal subdermal venule (0.3 mm) was joined to the proximal subdermal venule postoperatively. The finger survived completely without congestion (**Fig. 2**).

Case 2: Fascicular Turnover Flap for Facial Nerve Defect

A 68-year-old woman had a larger left parotid tumor, pleomorphic adenoma, for 20 years. After an extirpation of the tumor, buccal branches of the facial nerve were resected. The nerve defect (3 cm) was repaired with a fascicular turnover flap from one of the distal buccal branch. Fascicular nerve anastomosis was performed with a 50 μm needle (12-0 Crown Jun suture material). This nerve flap had reverse-flow from the distal buccal branch, and all Schwann cells within the flap could survive to accept rapid nerve regeneration from the proximal nerve. The postoperative recovery of her facial nerve function was excellent. A few months after surgery, functional recovery occurred and the patient gained normal function at 1 year, postoperatively (**Fig. 3**).

Case 3: Lymphaticovenular Anastomosis for Obstructive Lymphedema

A 64-year-old woman had secondary lymphedema and complete brachial nerve palsy of the left upper arm for 11 years. Sixteen years ago, she received a mastectomy and radiation. Two lymphaticovenular anastomoses were performed at the forearm. There was remarkable improvement of the affected arm after surgery and the patient did not need postoperative compression and physiotherapy. It is thought that degenerated smooth muscle cells within the anastomosed lymphatics were regenerate because of surgical bypass effect and the arm regained the lymph-drainage function (**Fig. 4**).

Case 4: Silicon Mastitis with Deep Inferior Epigastric Perforator Adiposal Perforator-to-Perforator Flap

The major perforators from the deep inferior epigastric artery anatomically locate around the umbilicus. The size of these perforators is usually 0.5 to 0.8 mm, which can be anastomosed to the same size recipient vessels. The flap can be thinned with removal of fatty tissue in one stage (**Fig. 5**).

A 53-year-old woman with painful silicon mastitis was repaired by silicon removal and simultaneous DIEP adiposal flap transfer with a short pedicle. The pedicle perforators with or without T segment of the deep inferior epigastric artery were joined to the distal level of the lateral thoracic vessel. Postoperatively, the patient had regained normal shape and softness of breast and had no pain (**Fig. 6**).

DISCUSSION

Supermicrosurgical innovative technology developed new free tissue transfers, including distal phalangeal replantation, toe-tip or vascularized toenail transfers, partial auricular flap or concha flap for eyelid and tracheal loss, lymphaticovenular anastomosis for lymphedema, and vascularized appendix transfer for penile urethral loss. Also, the pedicle perforator or short pedicle of perforator flaps can be anastomosed to small (<1 mm) or large recipient vessels with this technique.

Supermicrosurgical lymphaticovenular anastomosis is a new topic for treatment of lymphedema. Based on the authors' more than 500 cases, the surgery with more than 10 anastomoses can be

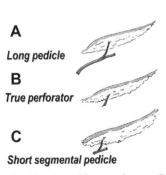

A

Long pedicle

B

True perforator

C

Short segmental pedicle

Fig. 1. The classification of free perforator flaps. (*A*) A long pedicle perforator flap. (*B*) Short T-segmental pedicle flap, which is useful as a flow-through flap. (*C*) A true perforator flap.

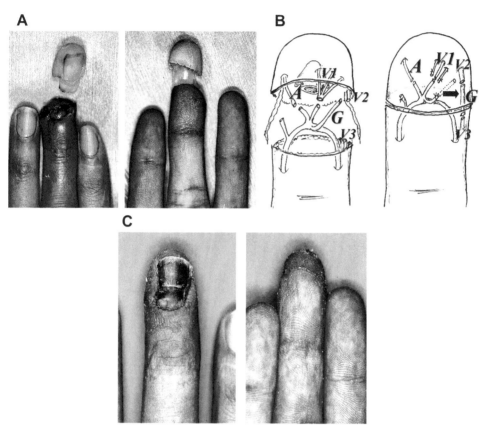

Fig. 2. (*A*) A 47-year-old man had an amputation of the left middle finger. (*B*) Under digital block, the proximal arteriole of digital artery (A) was anastomosed to the distal volar cutaneous venule (V1), and the distal ulnar venule (V2) was anastomosed to the proximal cutaneous vein (V3) with arteriolar graft (G) as drainage system. (*C*) At 2 months after surgery.

possible within 3 hours under local anesthesia. The result is dependent upon the number of anastomoses (more than 5 anastomoses in 1 limb is desirable), and stage of edema (early stage is the best). For severe edema cases resistant to left ventricle (LV) anastomosis, the authors confirm the effect of a free vascularized lymphoadipose flap with a smaller perforating vessel and lymphovenous anastomoses for establishment of the lymph drainage function. The authors are also trying prophylactic LV anastomosis simultaneous with cancer removal. The concept of this surgery is to preserve the normal drainage function of lymph smooth muscle cells, which seems to be the best method to prevent lymphedema. The next topic in lymphedema may be supermicrosurgical vascularized lymphoadipose flap and prophylactic LV anastomosis.

Another topic of supermicrosurgery is the introduction of nerve reconstructions. Peripheral nerves have rich vascular systems and all of those come from perforating vessels of perforator flaps.

Vascularized nerve flaps, such as the deep peroneal nerve flap and the lateral femoral cutaneous nerves, are now used for longer nerve gap and showing excellent motor and sensory recovery. Vascularization of nerve is always essential even in nerve transfer because survival of Schwann cells within a nerve flap is an important factor for nerve recovery. Vascularized cross-face nerve flap using an intraoral transfer of lateral femoral cutaneous nerve was proved to be a useful method for total removal of facial nerve. This method is indicated in the early stage of palsy. In addition, excellent functional recovery using fascicular turnover flap was reported for short nerve gap of facial and digital nerve reconstruction because this fascicular flap has reverse-flow blood circulation. Although supermicrosurgical anastomosis of single fascicle is difficult and needs some training, this concept and technique will be essential in the next phase of nerve reconstruction.

Regarding the recipient vessels for perforator-to-perforator flaps, many branches of temporal

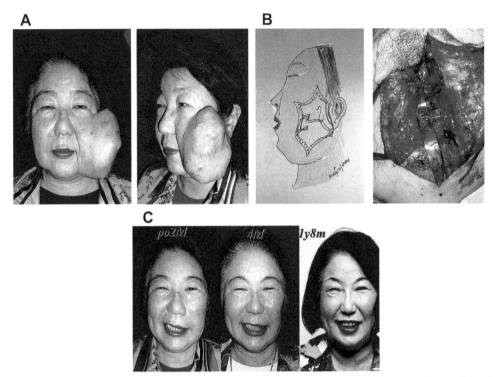

Fig. 3. (A) A larger pleomorphic adenoma for 20 years. (B) After an extirpation of the tumor, buccal branches of the facial nerve were resected. The nerve defect, of 3 cm, was repaired with fascicular turnover flap from the distal buccal branch. Fascicular nerve anastomosis was performed with 50 μm needle (12–0 Crown Jun suture material). (C) The postoperative recovery was excellent. At 2 months after surgery, functional recovery occurred and gained normal function within 1 year, postoperatively. Left, 2 months; middle, 4 months; right, 1 year and 8 months.

artery, facial artery, frontal artery, internal mammary artery, lateral thoracic artery, serratus muscle branch of the thoracodorsal system, radial artery, digital artery, anterior tibial artery, lateral and medial tarsal artery, and plantar digital artery were used. Vein grafts from the wrist volar aspect and foot dorsum are often used.

Free adiposal flap for facial and breast augmentation is the new topic in aesthetic supermicrosurgery. Based on the authors' more than 100 cases

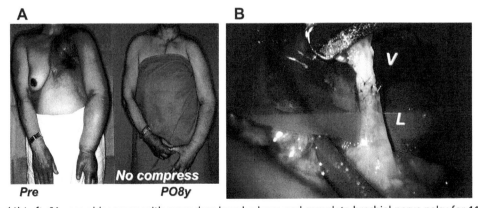

Fig. 4. (A) Left, 64-year-old woman with secondary lymphedema and complete brachial nerve palsy for 11 years. Sixteen years ago, she received mastectomy and radiation. Right, 8 years after surgery. Two lymphaticovenular anastomoses were performed at the forearm. There was remarkable improvement of the arm. The patient did not need postoperative compression and physiotherapy. The degenerated smooth muscle cells within anastomosed lymphatics might be regenerate because of bypass effect. (B) Lymphaticovenular anastomosis at the elbow fossa. L, lymphatic channel; V, venule.

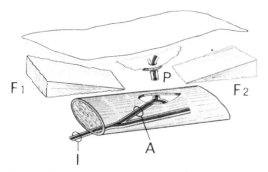

Fig. 5. Thin DIEP true perforator flap. The major perforators from the deep inferior epigastric artery are anatomically located around the umbilicus. The flap can be thinned with removal of fatty tissue in one stage. These perforators of DIEP flap can be anastomosed to the same size recipient vessels. (*From* Koshima I, et al. New microsurgical breast reconstruction using free PUP (paraumbilical perforator) adiposal flaps. Plast Reconstr Surg 2000;106:61–5; with permission.)

in 20 years, the potential of adiposal flap is greater than free fat injection and conventional dermal fat flap. This flap is indicated for any cases with a highly irradiated recipient, congenital hemifacial atrophy, and facial deformity after wide cancer removal. Adiposal flaps using DIEP, TAP, SCIP, and superficial inferior epigastric artery seem to be good donor candidates in young female patients. Also, intraoral transfer is the best approach for facial augmentation to avoid lateral bulkiness and postoperative drooping of the flap.

The advantages of these true perforator flaps include its simple operation, short time flap elevation, flaps can be obtained from anywhere in concealed areas, and it is a minimally invasive operation with less invasive donor-site morbidity. The disadvantages include their anatomic variation, the need for supermicrosurgical technique to dissect, and the technical difficulty for anastomosis with smaller vessels. These flaps are indicated for extremity reconstructions because

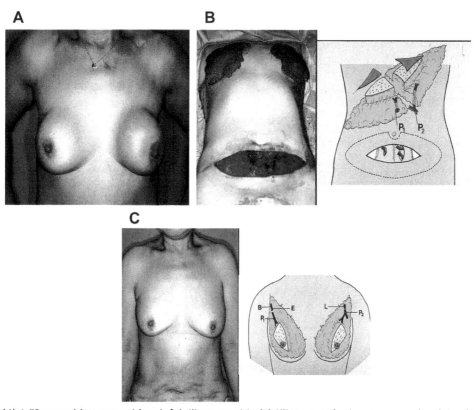

Fig. 6. (*A*) A 53-year-old woman with painful silicon mastitis. (*B*) Silicon prosthesis was removed and simultaneous DIEP adiposal flaps with short pedicle (P1, P2) were transferred. (*C*) Left, 2 years after surgery. The patient had regained normal shape and softness of breast and had no pain. Right, the pedicle perforators (P1, P2) were joined to the distal level of lateral thoracic vessel (B, right lateral thoracic artery; E, right lateral thoracic vein; L, left lateral thoracic vessel). (*From* Koshima I, et al. New microsurgical breast reconstruction using free PUP (paraumbilical perforator) adiposal flaps. Plast Reconstr Surg 2000;106:61–5; with permission.)

there are many recipient perforators of the same size as the flap perforators.

Technical tips for successful results include the use of duplicated vascular anastomoses using smaller recipient arteries and vein grafts; and flow-through vascular anastomosis using a T-shaped pedicle vessel, including perforator, assures double arterial inflow within a flap, and is indicated for ischemic extremities. The use of postoperative vasodilating drugs (prostaglandin E1) are recommended for successful results.

Finally, with supermicrosurgical techniques, many new flaps with a true perforator may be invented in the future. These flaps and vascularized tissues may be transferred without skin incision and sometimes flaps may be transferred under local anesthesia. New fields may be expected in all fields of surgery.

ACKNOWLEDGMENTS

I sincerely thank Dr Katsuyuki Urushibara, my coworker at Kawasaki Medical School, for his great contribution to the development of supermicrosurgery and the perforator flap. He died at the age of 44 by traffic accident on August 22, 2009.

REFERENCES

1. Koshima I. Microsurgery in the future: Introduction to supra-microsurgery and perforator flaps. Presented at the First International Course on Perforator Flap and Arterialized Skin Flaps. Special invited lecture. Gent, Belgium, June 13, 1997.
2. Yamano Y. Replantation of the amputated distal part of the fingers. J Hand Surg 1985;10:211.
3. Koshima I, Soeda S, Moriguchi T, et al. The use of arteriovenous anastomosis for replantation of the distal phalanx of the fingers. Plast Reconstr Surg 1992;89:710–4.
4. Koshima I, Itoh S, Takahashi Y, et al. Free vascularized nail graft under digital block. J Reconstr Microsurg 2001;17:599–601.
5. Koshima I, Inagawa K, Urushibara K, et al. Fingertip reconstructions using partial-toe transfers. Plast Reconstr Surg 2000;105:1666–74.
6. Koshima I, Inagawa K, Okuyama N, et al. Free vascularized appendix transfer for reconstruction of penile urethra with severe fibrosis. Plast Reconstr Surg 1999;103:964–9.
7. Fujino T, Harashina T, Nakajima T. Free skin flap from the retroauricular region to the nose. Plast Reconstr Surg 1976;57:338.
8. Parkhouse N, Evance D. Reconstruction of the ala of the nose using a composite free flap from the pinna. Br J Plast Surg 1985;38:306–13.
9. Shenaq SM, Dinh TA, Spira M. Nasal ala reconstruction with an ear helix free flap. J Reconstr Microsurg 1989;5:63–7.
10. Pribaz JJ, Falco N. Nasal reconstruction with auricular microvascular transplant. Ann Plast Surg 1993; 31:289–97.
11. Tanaka Y, Tajima S, Tsujiguchi K, et al. Microvascular reconstruction of nose and ear defects using composite auricular free flaps. Ann Plast Surg 1996;36:298–302.
12. Koshima I, Urushibara K, Okuyama H, et al. Ear helix flap for reconstruction of total loss of the upper eyelid. Br J Plast Surg 1999;52:314–6.
13. Koshima I, Umeda N, Moriguchi T, et al. A full-thickness chondrocutaneous flap from the auricular concha for repair of tracheal defects. Plast Reconstr Surg 1997;99:1887–93.
14. Koshima I, Inagawa K, Urushibara K, et al. Combined submental flap with toe web for reconstruction of the lip with oral commissure. Br J Plast Surg 2000;53:616–9.
15. Koshima I, Okumoto K, Umeda N, et al. Free vascularized deep peroneal nerve grafts. J Reconstr Microsurg 1996;12:131–41.
16. Koshima I, Narushima M, Mihara M, et al. Fascicular turnover flap for nerve gaps. J Plast Reconstr Aesthet Surg 2010;63(6):1008–14.
17. O'Brien BM, Sykes PJ, Threlfall GN, et al. Microlymphaticovenous anastomoses for obstructive lymphedema. Plast Reconstr Surg 1977;60: 197–211.
18. Koshima I, Inagawa K, Urushibara K, et al. Supermicrosurgical lymphaticovenular anastomosis for the treatment of lymphedema in the upper extremities. J Reconstr Microsurg 2000;16:437–42.
19. Koshima I, Nanba Y, Tsutsui T, et al. Long-term follow-up after lymphaticovenular anastomosis for lymphedema in the legs. J Reconstr Microsurg 2003;19:209–15.
20. Koshima I, Fujitsu M, Ushio S, et al. Flow-through anterior thigh flaps with a short pedicle for reconstruction of lower leg and foot defects. Plast Reconstr Surg 2005;115(1):155–62.
21. Koshima I, Inagawa K, Jitsuiki Y, et al. Scarpa's adipofascial flap for repair of wide scalp defects. Ann Plast Surg 1998;102:88–92.
22. Koshima I, Inagawa K, Urushibara K, et al. Paraumbilical perforator flap without deep inferior epigastric vessels. Plast Reconstr Surg 1998;102:1052–7.
23. Koshima I, Inagawa K, Yamamoto M, et al. New microsurgical breast reconstruction using free PUP (paraumbilical perforator) adiposal flaps. Plast Reconstr Surg 2000;106:61–5.
24. Koshima I, Inagawa K, Urushibara K, et al. One-stage facial contour augmentation with intraoral transfer of a paraumbilical perforator adiposal flap. Plast Reconstr Surg 2001;108:988–94.

25. Koshima I, Tsutsui T, Takahashi Y, et al. Free gluteal artery perforator flap with a short, small perforator. Ann Plast Surg 2003;51:200–4.

26. Inoue T, Kobayashi M, Harashina T. Finger pulp reconstruction with a free sensory medial plantar flap. Br J Plast Surg 1988;41:657.

27. Ishikura N, Heshiki T, Tsukada S. The use of a free medialis pedis flap for resurfacing skin defects of the hand and digits: results in five cases. Plast Reconstr Surg 1995;95:100.

28. Lee HB, Tark KC, Rah DK, et al. Pulp reconstruction of fingers with very small sensate medial plantar free flap. Plast Reconstr Surg 1998;101:999.

29. Koshima I, Urushibara K, Inagawa K, et al. Free medial plantar perforator flaps for the resurfacing of finger and foot defects. Plast Reconstr Surg 2001;107:1753–7.

30. Koshima I. Short pedicle superficial inferior epigastric artery adiposal flap: new anatomical findings and the use of this flap for reconstruction of facial contour. Plast Reconstr Surg 2005;116(4):1091 7.

Index

Note: Page numbers of article titles are in **boldface** type.

A

Abdomen, regional overview of, 659, 660
Abdominal flaps, lower, in breast reconstruction, 641–644
Angiography, 3-D, advantages of, 555–557
 anatomic technique, 554, 555
 demonstration in layer-by-layer process using, 554, 555
 for reconstruction of arterial system, 555–558
 for reconstruction of pelvic bones, 555, 558
 in injection studies, 554, 556
 of anatomy of perforator flaps, 555–558
 of peroneal artery and fibula, 559
 of vascular anatomy, 554
 CT. See *CT angiography.*
 MR. See *MR angiography.*
Angiosomes, of source vessels, vascular territories of body and, 553, 556
Arm, lateral, flap harvesting from, 668
 perforator flaps of, 668, 669
 vascular anatomy of, 668–672
Artery(ies), anterior intercostal, perforator flaps, 658
 circumflex scapular, perforator flaps, 662
 deep inferior epigastric, perforator flaps, 660, 661, 662
 dorsal intercostal, perforator flaps, 662, 663
 dorsal metacarpal, first, perforator flaps, 672, 673
  reverse, perforator flaps, 674
  second, perforator flaps, 673, 674
 dorsal scapular, perforator flaps, 661, 662
 epigastric, deep inferior, vascular anatomy of, 581
 intercostal, perforator flap, in breast reconstruction, 649, 650
 internal mammary, perforator flaps, 657, 658
 lateral intercostal, perforator flaps, 658, 659
 lumbar, perforator flaps, 663
 occipital, perforator flaps, 635, 636
 of upper extremity, 561, 563
 peroneal, and fibula, 3-D angiography of, 559
 posterior interosseous, perforator flaps, 669, 670
 proximal radial, perforator flaps, 672
 radial, perforator flaps, 671, 672
 subcostal, perforator flaps, 663
 submental, perforator flap, anatomy of, 629
  background of, 629
  planning and surgical dissection of, 629, 630
 superficial temporal, perforator flaps. See *Perforator flap(s), superficial temporal artery-based.*
 superior epigastric, perforator flaps, 659, 660
 supraclavicular, perforator flaps. See *Perforator flap(s), supraclavicular artery-based.*
 thoracodorsal, perforator flaps, 658, 659
 ulnar, perforator flaps of, 670, 671
Axial flaps, 572
Axial pattern flaps, from trunk, 655, 656

B

Back, upper, coverage of defects of, 656, 660–663
Blood supply, regional, of trunk, 656
Blood vessels, recipient, for perforator flap, selection and preparation of, 602
Breast, and trunk, defects on, propeller flaps for, 621, 622
 reconstruction of, abdomen-based microsurgical, preoperative imaging techniques for perforator selection in, **581–591**
  autogenous tissues for, 612
  deep inferior epigastric artery perforator flap in, 642, 643, 687
  gluteal artery perforator flaps for, 644–647
  intercostal artery perforator flap for, 649, 650
  lower abdominal flaps for, 641–644
  pedicled perforator flaps for, 647, 648
  perforator flaps in, 575–576, **641–654**
   preoperative imaging for, 650–652
  superficial inferior epigastric flap, and deep inferior epigastric artery perforator flap for, 642, 643, 645
  superficial inferior epigastric flap in, 643, 644
  thoracodorsal artery perforator flaps for, 648, 649
  transverse rectus abdominis myocutaneous flap in, 641, 642
Buttock, defects of, propeller flaps for, 622–624
 vascular anatomy of, 568
Buttock region, perforator flaps in, 576

C

Carotid artery, external, principal branches of, 562
Chest, regional overview of, 657–659
Chest wall, perforator flaps in, 576
Chimeric flaps, 594
Color duplex ultrasound, clinical studies with, 583
 for information on perforators, 582–587
 introduction of, 583, 584
 sample report, 582, 583
 technique of, 582–587

Clin Plastic Surg 37 (2010) 691–694
doi:10.1016/S0094-1298(10)00103-3

plasticsurgery.theclinics.com

Color (*continued*)
  versus CT angiography, for preoperative mapping of perforators, 587
Computed tomographic angiography, in breast reconstruction, 651, 652
CT angiography, accuracy of, for locating perforators, 584, 585
  and operative time, 585–587
  in breast reconstruction, 651, 652
  technique of, 584, 586, 587
  versus color duplex ultrasound, for preoperative mapping for perforators, 587
Cutaneous free flaps, 572

D

Doppler ultrasound, to locate perforators, 581, 582

F

Facial nerve defect, fascicular turnover flap for, 684, 686
FAP flap, anatomy of, 630, 631
  background of, 630
  planning and surgical dissection of, 631, 632
  special considerations for, 632, 633
Fasciocutaneous flaps, peninsular, 615, 616
Fibula, and peroneal artery, 3-D angiography of, 559
Forearm, radial, perforator flaps of, 671, 672
  ulnar, perforator flaps of, 670, 671
  vascular territories of, 667–669
Free flaps, cutaneous, 572

G

Gluteal artery perforator flaps, inferior, in breast reconstruction, 644–647
  superior, in breast reconstruction, 646, 647

H

Hand, intrinsic flaps of, 672–674
  volar, integument of, angiogram of, 563, 564
Head and neck, cutaneous vasculature of, 558–562
  perforator flaps for, 574, 575

I

Imaging techniques, preoperative, for perforator selection in abdomen-based microsurgical breast reconstruction, **581–591**
Injection studies, in 3-D angiography, 554, 556
Innervated free flaps, 594

K

Kite flap, proximally pedicled, 672, 673

L

Lower extremity, cutaneous vasculature of, 566–569
  integument of, 567
  perforator flaps use in, 577
Lumbar-subcostal region, coverage of defects of, 663
Lymphaticovenular anastomosis, for obstructive lymphedema, 684, 686
Lymphedema, obstructive, lymphaticovenular anastomosis for, 684, 686

M

Malignant melanoma, excision of, propeller flaps for closure of chest wall following, 621, 622
Medial maleolus, loss of, with exposure of tibia, 618
Microsurgical tissue transfers, 611
MR angiography, advantages of, 588, 589
  disadvantages of, 588
  for perforator-based breast reconstruction, 587–590
  in breast reconstruction, 652
  techniques and clinical studies using, 588–590
Muscle flaps, from trunk, choice of, 655, 656

P

Pelvic reconstruction, perforator flaps in, 576
Perforator flap(s), advancement flap, 601, 602
  anatomic area, CT imaging of, 595
  anatomic basis of, **553–570**
  anatomy of, 3-D angiography of, 555–558
  and supermicrosurgery, **683, 689**
  anterior intercostal artery, 658
  circumflex scapular artery, 662
  clinical benefits of, 627, 628
  complications and limitations of, 602–604
  current status of, 574
  deep inferior epigastric artery, 660–662
    and superficial inferior epigastric flap, in breast reconstruction, 642, 643, 645
    in breast reconstruction, 642, 643, 687
  design modifications and refinements for, 594
  design of, angiosome concept of, 573
    considerations in, 628, 629
  disadvantages of, 581
  dissection of, deep fascia and, 597, 598
    incision and approach for, 595–597
    intramuscular, 598–601
    main pedicle and, 600, 601
    operative technique for, 595
  distal ulnar, 671
  dorsal intercostal artery, 662, 663
  dorsal scapular artery, 661, 662
  evolution of, 627
  facial artery-based, 629–639

first dorsal metacarpal artery, 672, 673
for head and neck, 574, 575
for upper extremity, 575
from trunk, 656
general considerations and, 573, 574
gluteal artery, inferior, in breast reconstruction, 644–647
    superior, in breast reconstruction, 646, 647
historical perspective on, 571–573
imaging for dissection of, 594, 595
in head and neck, source vessels for, 628
in reconstruction of breast, 575, 576, **641–654**
in upper extremity, **667–676**
intercostal artery, in breast reconstruction, 649, 650
internal mammary artery, 657, 658
    anatomy of, 638
    background of, 638
    planning and surgical dissection in, 638
    special considerations in, 638, 639
lateral arm, 668, 669
lateral intercostal artery, 658, 659
lumbar artery, 663
muscle, 612
    "big four" of, 610
    integration into community-based private practice, **607–614**
new classification of, 683, 684
nomenclature of, 569, 570
    and classification of, 572, 573
occipital artery-based, 635, 636
pedicled, in breast reconstruction, 647, 648
    in head and neck, **627–640**
        clinical applications of, 629
    in trunk, **655–665**
pedicled anterolateral thigh, 677–680
perforator vessel dissection, technical tips for safe, applicable to all flaps, **593–606**
posterior interosseous artery, 669, 670
preoperative imaging of, 603
preoperative planning for, 593, 594
proximal radial artery, 672
proximal ulnar, 671
radial artery, 671, 672
reverse dorsal metacarpal artery, 674
rotation flap, 601
second dorsal metacarpal artery, 673, 674
subcostal artery, 663
submental artery, anatomy of, 629
    background of, 629
    planning and surgical dissection of, 629, 630
superficial temporal artery-based, anatomy of, 633
    background of, 633
    planning and surgical dissection of, 633–635
    special considerations in, 635
superior epigastric artery, 659, 660

supraclavicular artery-based, anatomy of, 636
    background of, 636
    planning and surgical dissection of, 636, 637
    special considerations in, 637, 638
thoracodorsal artery, 658, 659
    in breast reconstruction, 648, 649
to-perforator flap, deep inferior epigastric perforator adiposal, in silicon mastitis, 684, 687
transposition flap, 602
ulnar artery, 670, 671
venous drainage of, 573
venous system and, 602–604
where do they fit in our armamentarium?, **571–579**
Perforators, Doppler ultrasound to locate, 581, 582
forms of, deep fascia and integrument, 607–609
information on, color duplex ultrasound for, 582–587
locating of, CT angiography for, 584, 585
of anterior thigh, 568
of body, 557–561
of lower leg, 569
preoperative mapping of, CT angiography versus color duplex ultrasound for, 587
vessel dissection, technical tips for safe, applicable to all perforator flaps, **593–606**
vessels, ultrasonographic evaluation of, 595
Perineal reconstruction, perforator flaps in, 576
Phalangeal replantation, distal, 684, 685
Propeller flap, based distally for distal lower limb reconstruction, 616
concept of, **615–626**
description of, 615, 616
for closure of anterior chest wall following malignant melanoma excision, 621, 622
for defects of buttock, 622–624
for defects on trunk and breast, 621, 622
for distal lower limb defects, flap design for, 617
    indications for, 619
    raising flap for, 617–619
    rotation and inset of, 619
    surgical technique for, 617–624
for upper limb defects, 619–621
indications for, 623, 624
islanding of, 616, 617
safety and reliability of, 624
single pedicle, 616
to cover defect resulting from basal cell carcinoma, 623

S

Silicon mastitis, deep inferior epigastric perforator adiposal perforator-to-perforator flap in, 684, 687
Soft tissue reconstruction, materials and methods for, 609, 610
results of, 609, 610

Superficial inferior epigastric flap, and deep inferior
   epigastric artery perforator flap, in breast
   reconstruction, 642–645
   in breast reconstruction, 643, 644
Supermicrosurgery, history of, 683
   perforator flaps and, **683–689**
      technique of, case reports of, 684
Supramicrosurgery. See *Supermicrosurgery.*

T

Thigh, anterolateral, pedicled perforator flaps of,
   677–680
Thigh flap, for degloving injury of hindfoot, 607, 608
   pedicled anterolateral, arc of rotation of, 679, 680
      design of, 677, 678
      prevention of complications of, 680
      vascular anatomy of, 677, 678
      versatility of, **677–681**
Thin flaps, 594
Thoracodorsal artery perforator flaps, in breast
   reconstruction, 648, 649
Thumb, vascular anatomy of, 672
Thumb flap, dorsal ulnar, 672, 673
Tibia, exposure of, loss of medial malleolus with, 618
Transverse rectus abdominis myocutaneous flap, in
   breast reconstruction, 641, 642
Trunk, and breast, defects on, propeller flaps
   for, 621, 622
   cutaneous vasculature of, 563–566
   pedicled perforator flaps in, **655–665**

reconstruction of, perforator flaps in, 576
regional blood supply of, 656

U

Ulna, distal, perforator flaps of, 671
   dorsal, thumb flap of, 672, 673
   proximal, perforator flaps of, 671
Ultrasound, color duplex. See *Color duplex
   ultrasound.*
   Doppler, to locate perforators, 581, 582
Upper extremity, arteries of, 561, 563
   cutaneous vasculature of, 561–564
   integument of, angiogram of, 561–563
   perforator flaps in, 575, **667–676**
Upper limbs, defects of, propeller flap for, 619–621

V

Vascular anatomy, 3-D angiography of, 554
Vascular pedicle, long, 611
Vascular territories of body, 553–555, 560, 561
   and angiosomes of source vessels of, 553, 556
   and source arteries supplying perforators,
      557, 559
Vasculature, cutaneous, historical perspective
   on, 553
      of head and neck, 558–562
      of lower extremity, 566–569
      of trunk, 563–566
      of upper extremity, 561–564

United States Postal Service

Statement of Ownership, Management, and Circulation
(All Periodicals Publications Except Requestor Publications)

1. Publication Title	2. Publication Number	3. Filing Date
Clinics in Plastic Surgery	0 0 6 - 5 3 3 0	9/15/10

4. Issue Frequency	5. Number of Issues Published Annually	6. Annual Subscription Price
Jan, Apr, Jul, Oct	4	$384.00

7. Complete Mailing Address of Known Office of Publication (*Not printer*) (*Street, city, county, state, and ZIP+4®*)

Elsevier Inc.
360 Park Avenue South
New York, NY 10010-1710

Contact Person
Stephen Bushing
Telephone (Include area code)
215-239-3688

8. Complete Mailing Address of Headquarters or General Business Office of Publisher (*Not printer*)

Elsevier Inc., 360 Park Avenue South, New York, NY 10010-1710

9. Full Names and Complete Mailing Addresses of Publisher, Editor, and Managing Editor (*Do not leave blank*)

Publisher (*Name and complete mailing address*)

Kim Murphy, Elsevier, Inc., 1600 John F. Kennedy Blvd. Suite 1800, Philadelphia, PA 19103-2899

Editor (*Name and complete mailing address*)

Barbara Cohen-Kligerman, Elsevier, Inc., 1600 John F. Kennedy Blvd. Suite 1800, Philadelphia, PA 19103-2899

Managing Editor (*Name and complete mailing address*)

Catherine Bewick, Elsevier, Inc., 1600 John F. Kennedy Blvd. Suite 1800, Philadelphia, PA 19103-2899

10. Owner (*Do not leave blank. If the publication is owned by a corporation, give the name and address of the corporation immediately followed by the names and addresses of all stockholders owning or holding 1 percent or more of the total amount of stock. If not owned by a corporation, give the names and addresses of the individual owners. If owned by a partnership or other unincorporated firm, give its name and address as well as those of each individual owner. If the publication is published by a nonprofit organization, give its name and address.*)

Full Name	Complete Mailing Address
Wholly owned subsidiary of	4520 East-West Highway
Reed/Elsevier, US holdings	Bethesda, MD 20814

11. Known Bondholders, Mortgagees, and Other Security Holders Owning or Holding 1 Percent or More of Total Amount of Bonds, Mortgages, or Other Securities. If none, check box ☐ None

Full Name	Complete Mailing Address
N/A	

12. Tax Status (*For completion by nonprofit organizations authorized to mail at nonprofit rates*) (Check one)
The purpose, function, and nonprofit status of this organization and the exempt status for federal income tax purposes:
☐ Has Not Changed During Preceding 12 Months
☐ Has Changed During Preceding 12 Months (*Publisher must submit explanation of change with this statement*)

PS Form 3526, September 2007 (Page 1 of 3 (Instructions Page 3)) PSN 7530-01-000-9931 PRIVACY NOTICE: See our Privacy policy in www.usps.com

13. Publication Title	14. Issue Date for Circulation Data Below
Clinics in Plastic Surgery	July 2010

15. Extent and Nature of Circulation			Average No. Copies Each Issue During Preceding 12 Months	No. Copies of Single Issue Published Nearest to Filing Date
a. Total Number of Copies (*Net press run*)			2263	2150
b. Paid Circulation (By Mail and Outside the Mail)	(1)	Mailed Outside-County Paid Subscriptions Stated on PS Form 3541. (*Include paid distribution above nominal rate, advertiser's proof copies, and exchange copies*)	925	903
	(2)	Mailed In-County Paid Subscriptions Stated on PS Form 3541 (*Include paid distribution above nominal rate, advertiser's proof copies, and exchange copies*)		
	(3)	Paid Distribution Outside the Mails Including Sales Through Dealers and Carriers, Street Vendors, Counter Sales, and Other Paid Distribution Outside USPS®	558	522
	(4)	Paid Distribution by Other Classes Mailed Through the USPS (e.g. First-Class Mail®)		
c. Total Paid Distribution (*Sum of 15b (1), (2), (3), and (4)*) ▶			1483	1425
d. Free or Nominal Rate Distribution (By Mail and Outside the Mail)	(1)	Free or Nominal Rate Outside-County Copies Included on PS Form 3541	73	68
	(2)	Free or Nominal Rate In-County Copies Included on PS Form 3541		
	(3)	Free or Nominal Rate Copies Mailed at Other Classes Through the USPS (e.g. First-Class Mail)		
	(4)	Free or Nominal Rate Distribution Outside the Mail (Carriers or other means)		
e. Total Free or Nominal Rate Distribution (Sum of 15d (1), (2), (3) and (4)) ▶			73	68
f. Total Distribution (Sum of 15c and 15e) ▶			1556	1493
g. Copies not Distributed (See instructions to publishers #4 (page #3)) ▶			707	657
h. Total (Sum of 15f and g) ▶			2263	2150
i. Percent Paid (15c divided by 15f times 100) ▶			95.31%	95.45%

16. Publication of Statement of Ownership

☐ If the publication is a general publication, publication of this statement is required. Will be printed
   in the **October 2010** issue of this publication.   ☐ Publication not required

17. Signature and Title of Editor, Publisher, Business Manager, or Owner	Date
Stephen R. Bushing Stephen R. Bushing – Fulfillment/Inventory Specialist	September 15, 2010

I certify that all information furnished on this form is true and complete. I understand that anyone who furnishes false or misleading information on this form or who omits material or information requested on the form may be subject to criminal sanctions (including fines and imprisonment) and/or civil sanctions (including civil penalties).

PS Form 3526, September 2007 (Page 2 of 3)

Moving?

Make sure your subscription moves with you!

To notify us of your new address, find your **Clinics Account Number** (located on your mailing label above your name), and contact customer service at:

Email: journalscustomerservice-usa@elsevier.com

800-654-2452 (subscribers in the U.S. & Canada)
314-447-8871 (subscribers outside of the U.S. & Canada)

Fax number: 314-447-8029

Elsevier Health Sciences Division
Subscription Customer Service
3251 Riverport Lane
Maryland Heights, MO 63043

*To ensure uninterrupted delivery of your subscription, please notify us at least 4 weeks in advance of move.

ELSEVIER

Printed and bound by CPI Group (UK) Ltd, Croydon, CR0 4YY

03/10/2024

01040357-0017